VIBRATING YOUTH *On a budget!*

Affordable things to do in your 20s, 30s and 40s,
to look fabulous in your 50s, 60s, 70s and beyond.

By

Toni Ann Johnson

To my mother Vera P. Johnson, who gave me good genes and good sense.

Table Of Contents

INTRODUCTION

People tell me I look young, *really* young, for my age. They have for sometime now, since my 20s, and it continues today now that I'm 46. For this, I have a number of factors like good genes, and a little melanin to thank, but I also have my mother who still looks startlingly young at an age I'm forbidden to reveal. Much of what I know, I learned from her.

My mother told me she was "21-plus" from the time I began to wonder about her age until I was 12 years old. Every year I would ask, "Plus *what,* Mommy?"

And she'd refuse to answer.

"But Mo-om, you were 21-plus *last* year, and the year before that," I'd whine. "You can't be the same thing every year."

Mom's birthday is just a week after mine. The summer I turned 12, once again, I wanted to know which year it was for her. We were having breakfast. Her face was hidden behind the morning newspaper. She lowered it to frown at me. "A woman who will tell her age will tell anything." She disappeared behind the paper again.

"What's *that* supposed to mean?" I demanded.

Once again, she lowered her paper. This time she leaned closer to my face and spoke through clenched teeth. "It means: *None of your business*."

Mom was scary. And the fact that I was never going to get an answer couldn't be clearer. But it *was* my business as far as I was concerned. So I snooped; went into her purse and found her driver's license. It would be years before I'd admit that I knew her secret. And to this day, I'm forbidden to tell anyone.

My mother was and still is a beautiful lady. She's always looked quite a bit younger than she is. To this day, she will not tell her age and has, in fact, *never* told me (or anyone else that I know of, except my father). If I hadn't seen it on her license, it's very possible that I'd still be wondering.

Recently we discussed taking a trip abroad together, which meant she would have to renew her passport. She told me it was going to take her a few weeks to make time to get up to the town where she would fill out the application for renewal. I told her she could do it at her local post office. She was quiet for a moment and then said, "Well, I prefer not to do that."

Why? She didn't want the people in her small town to know her real age. That's my mother: beautiful, vain as they come and pleased to keep people thinking she's much younger than she is.

Though people think I'm a lot younger than my real age as well, unfortunately I didn't inherit mom's air of mystery. Sometimes I have a big mouth. And I quite enjoy seeing the shock on people's faces and hearing them say, "Wow! You don't look it! What's your secret?!" I also love how they really listen when I begin to share that secret.

It was several years ago that I began to realize that there was, indeed, something a bit unusual about how young I looked. When I was 30, a doctor I hadn't seen before seemed shocked to learn that I was over 20. When joining a new gym at age 33, the guy signing me up asked if I'd need to have a parent co-sign the contract.

The event that really confirmed it for me, though, was when I traveled to Ghana at age 37 to write about a group of high school students who were on an educational excursion there, and one of the kids thought I was still in college. I told her, "No, I'm old."

"Please," she said, eyeing me. "Old. You're not even close to 25."

When she found out my real age she looked horrified. She actually recoiled. Her mouth fell open, "You're a mutant," she shrieked.

I took it as a compliment. A mutant. Ha! Maybe I am. I'm going to teach you to be one, too!

In this case, a "mutant" is a person who vibrates youth. What does it mean to "vibrate youth?" Hopefully the rest of the book will clarify that, but for now, here's what I'd like you to consider: When I speak of "vibrating," I'm talking about the energy or frequency at which something exists. For example, the energy of a healthy, living, green plant is much different from that of a dried out, dead plant. The energy of a brand new car is different from the energy of an old, beat-up, dirty car. In this case, we're talking about you and how you look, act and feel. My goal is share with you some tools that will help you attain your healthiest, happiest, clearest, most beautiful energy. You will be wiser, something that usually comes with age, but as you begin to cultivate a healthier, lovelier energy, you'll emit a glow that results from radiating at your best frequency. This is what it means to vibrate youth.

RETURNING THE BODY TO ITS PUREST STATE AND MAINTAINING IT

You know how when you've been living in a house or apartment for a long time and you accumulate a lot of junk and your closets get filled, dust settles in places, and the paint looks dirty and old? Your place *feels* old when that happens. The energy feels stagnant and perhaps, without being conscious of it, you feel a little sluggish or stuck, too.

Then one day (hopefully!) you've had enough and you decide to do a serious deep cleaning and sprucing up. Maybe you throw out a bunch of junk, vacuum or sweep under the bed, organize your files, clean the refrigerator, wash the walls, or put up a new coat of paint. When you're done, your old place has new energy; it's brighter, fresher and you feel better about living there.

My theory is that this kind of revitalization can apply to our bodies as well.

We've all heard about Feng Shui and the idea that energy flows better in our homes when things are arranged favorably and clutter is cleared away. Isn't it possible that our body's energy flows better when we clear out its clutter, too? If your colon is sluggish, there's plaque built up in your teeth, dead skin layered on your body, calluses on your feet, gunk under your toenails—you get the idea—you will feel clogged, weighed down, dull and maybe even a bit older than you should.

But if you cleanse your colon, scrub your skin, scrape your calluses and clean your nails and teeth out, you will feel lighter, fresher, revitalized.

Some cultures believe that cleansing the body has deeper spiritual benefits. I'm a regular at a Korean Day Spa in Los Angeles where women scrub from head to toe and remove toxins in the sauna, steam room, and by sitting in special hot and cold pools. It is believed that these cleansing rituals leave one prepared to attract more auspicious circumstances.

This may sound absurd to one who hasn't experienced it, but I have. I'm a believer in cleansing inside and out. I did "The Master Cleanse" fast while in my late 20s, for 9 days. You're supposed to do it for 10, but I didn't make it. Nevertheless, by the 9th day, I looked like a new person! My skin glowed, my eyes were bright, I was thinner, I radiated peace and happiness. I looked 10 years younger.

All that I'd done was empty my intestines completely and replace all the junk I'd been eating with nothing but water, lemon juice, maple syrup, cayenne pepper and tea. All that liquid and the break in eating solid food had literally transformed me. The difference in my appearance was remarkable, so remarkable that as a result, I was inspired to learn more about natural approaches to health and beauty.

I wouldn't recommend The Master Cleanse for weight loss. It does, of course, result in weight loss, but when normal eating resumes, you're likely to gain the weight back. But there were physical and mental benefits that I wouldn't have believed in had I not experienced them myself. It's quite possible that I'd have achieved the same results by drinking nothing but water for nine days, but I don't think I would have lasted as long on water alone. There's plenty of controversy around the Master Cleanse and many of the claims it makes have been widely dismissed. However, its positive effects on me, inside and out, got my attention and changed my life. That fast was the beginning of my journey toward a lifestyle wherein I'd use natural approaches to renewing my body and spirit.

Before I continue, I want to be clear that when I speak of "cleansing the colon," I mean the complete emptying of the intestines. I'm *not* referring to removing the so-called "mucoid plaque" that the purveyors of colon cleansers speak of.

According to medical doctors, there is no such thing as mucoid plaque, which has been described as old waste "lining" the colon. Dr. Ed Frielander, a pathologist who published a research paper on the web called "Ed's Guide to Alternative Therapies," says, "I have opened hundreds of colons and never seen anything like toxic bowel settlement."

The lining of the colon is similar to the lining of the mouth. Old waste does not stick to it. As my sister, Dr. Hillary Johnson, an internist, explains: *the colon doesn't get "dirty."* However, if you don't eat properly, the intestines may take longer to eliminate waste. Ideally, the bowels are emptied each day or every other day, though "normal" varies from person to person.

I'll discuss cleansing and fasting more later, but for now let me say that *long-term* fasting requires supervision and is not something I recommend. Most doctors don't advocate fasting and will likely discourage you from doing it. My friend Jill injured herself on the Master Cleanse, and ended up in the hospital after damaging the lining of her stomach. So if you decide to do a protracted fast, please see a doctor first and make sure there are no underlying medical issues that make the process dangerous for you. I was fortunate not to have suffered adverse health issues, but there can be risks.

My advice is to do brief fasts of 1 to 2 days, either on the Master Cleanse or juice fasting, a few times a year. And all during the year eat more fruits, vegetables, whole grains, nuts and legumes. Let these "whole foods," which are also high in fiber, make up the majority of your diet. They will help your colon function efficiently, because high fiber foods assist the intestines with elimination.

To jumpstart your path to vibrating youth, is to get yourself clean and clear, inside and out. This is what I mean my returning your body to its purest state. The goal is to get back to square one, before your body was polluted with gunk and junk. A short fast will clean you out on the inside. A body scrub will renew you on the outside.

Exfoliating the skin to reveal the new skin underneath is another thing that will help you look and feel younger. Our skin regenerates itself, shedding dead skin cells and revealing the newer cells, but as the skin gets older that process slows down. Exfoliating will help your skin look younger as you age, because it assists in the regenerative process.

As I mentioned, I'm a frequent visitor to a Korean spa in Los Angeles. Sloughing off dead skin to reveal the new skin underneath is one of the things encouraged there. They use hand-sized exfoliating pads and I've been shocked at how much skin rolls off my body when it's scrubbed with them. Afterwards, my skin looks fresh and youthful as if years have been removed from it.

You don't need to go to a spa to do achieve this, though. In fact, most of what I'm going to suggest in this book is designed to be inexpensive.

You can exfoliate with a loofah or a body brush or even some sea salt mixed with olive oil. However you choose to do it, be sure to remove old skin and reveal the new regularly. Do a good scrub at least every couple of months and always be sure to moisturize after exfoliating. Use sunscreen if you'll be outside in daylight.

Another thing that helps to keep the body clean and pure is something I've been doing since my early 30s, which is flossing my teeth every single day. Yes, *every* day.

Think about it—if you have stuff in your teeth that hardens into plaque and sits there, nothing good can come from that. Clean it out. If you don't, bacteria build up occurs and eventually that can seep into your bloodstream.

An article published by the American Academy of Periodontology states: "Researchers have found evidence that the amount of bacteria in subgingival plaques, the deep plaques in periodontal pockets and around the teeth, may contribute to an individual's risk of a heart attack, according to two studies appearing in the *Journal of Periodontology*. These studies further researchers' understanding that periodontal bacteria may increase the risk for heart disease."

Poor dental health has been linked to heart attack, stroke and diabetes. It may seem like a leap to say that there's a relationship between youth and flossing, but if flossing can help prevent heart disease, stroke and diabetes, it does something to promote good health, which, as I see it, is anti-aging.

Recent studies have suggested that periodontal disease is linked to Alzheimer's Disease, so there is actually some evidence to indicate that flossing can be beneficial to one's brain. And if that doesn't persuade you to floss, how about the idea of losing your teeth? That is a guaranteed path to looking like a granny! Joking aside, daily flossing helps to reduce the toxins that enter our system. I believe that reducing those toxins, in turn, helps to delay the aging process.

As you endeavor to keep your insides clean, your teeth free of plaque and your skin exfoliated, it's not a bad idea to keep your nails and toe nails clean, as well. This, too, will help to reduce the number of germs and toxins entering your body. According to an article called "5 Frightening Truths about the Dirt Under Your Fingernails (and his)" by Sandra Jio, your nails may be harboring bacteria that make you sick. Since no good can come from *that* better to clean it out. As a matter of simple aesthetics, you are going to look better, cleaner, fresher and yes, even younger, when your nails are free of bacteria filled gunk.

Like your home and your car, *everything* looks and feels a bit newer when it's had a good cleaning, even you. As you begin keeping your body renewed, clean, and free of unnecessary toxins, inside and out, you will inevitably be radiating more youth.

MOM'S ONE-TWO COMBINATION:
BRUSH YOUR FACE and TAKE OMEGA 3's

BRUSH YOUR FACE

I live in Los Angeles and my mother lives in New York. During a visit when I was in my early 30s, she told me to take Omega 3 capsules and to "brush my skin" everyday with a toothbrush. She had recently begun do these things, she said, and she'd noticed a very positive difference in her skin. *Brush my skin with a toothbrush? What?* I thought it sounded crazy. "Yeah, yeah," I said, and never gave the advice a second thought. Just thought my mom was getting kookier as she was getting older.

Nearly two years went by before I had the opportunity to visit my mother again. I was stunned to see that her skin looked remarkable, much younger than it had during my previous visit. She told me that she'd been taking Omega 3's, fish oil and flaxseed oil, twice a day and *brushing her skin each day with a toothbrush.* This time I paid attention. I'll admit, the idea of brushing my skin with a toothbrush continued to sound crazy to me, but she looked so spectacular I was willing to hear more.

"Um, okay… A toothbrush, huh? What kind of toothbrush?"
"Just a regular, soft bristle toothbrush, that's all."

She showed me the one she was using. I asked how she did it and she told me to brush my face in a circular motion, all around, over and against the lines.

Mom discovered the skin brushing's anti-aging benefit by accident. She'd had acne prone skin as an adult, like I do. At one point, her pores were quite clogged and she decided to get a facial. During the treatment, the esthetician used a face brush on her skin and explained that regular skin brushing would help her pores remain clear. The brush was larger and softer than a toothbrush, but mom didn't feel like spending the money on a face brush, because she wasn't convinced that it would work. Instead, she opted to try a soft bristle toothbrush (less expensive), figuring it was similar enough to be just as effective. After brushing her face every day for a short while, she found that the regular toothbrush did, indeed, help to keep her pores clearer and reduce acne breakouts. After a year or so of brushing her face, she also found that the fine lines around her mouth and on her forehead had become less visible and soon she was brushing her entire face, not just the acne prone areas.

I've been doing it for over 10 years now and it's kept my skin looking like that of a much younger woman. I found that as I brush the skin on my face, in addition to exfoliating, I'm also massaging the facial muscles and manipulating the skin in ways that discourage the formation of lines.

For example, my forehead naturally produces horizontal lines because I raise my eyebrows repeatedly throughout day. I also have a habit of bringing the eyebrows together when I concentrate or frown. And I tend to get creases around my mouth from laughing and from sleeping on one side of my face. So I brush in a way that breaks up the pattern of those repetitive movements.

Here's my technique: I put soap or cleanser all over my face. Then, I add a bit to the toothbrush so that it will glide over the skin. On my forehead, I brush in a circle, clockwise and then counter clockwise, and also up and down over the places where there are lines from raising my eyebrows. Between the brows where frown lines can appear, I brush in a smaller circle, clockwise and counter clockwise. Around the laugh lines, I brush in circles, clockwise and counter clockwise along the length of the lines. Under my eyes, I brush softly from the outside in toward the bridge of the nose.

I remember this approach to battling eye wrinkles from modeling school when I was a teenager. Our teacher, Margo George, in Goshen, New York, told us to apply moisturizer with strokes from the side of the face in toward the nose. She said this would combat under-eye wrinkles and it's worked for me. For years, I've applied the same motion with the brush, gently brushing from the outside in.

I also go over the whole face, and neck (don't forget your neck!) brushing in small circles all around. Anyplace I see lines forming, I brush over that area, clockwise and counterclockwise. On the neck, I also brush up and down.

The brushing will exfoliate the skin and bring blood to the surface.

According to the website EARTHSAVERS, during face brushing: *"Exfoliation draws out impurities from the pores, stimulates circulation and brings oxygen and nutrients from the blood to feed and nourish skin cells."*

It's normal to look a bit red afterwards, if your skin is light, but the redness should disappear within a few minutes. This is similar to what microdermabrasion accomplishes, but, of course, it's far less costly and not as intense.

The makers of the Sonicare electric toothbrush have a product on the market that is similar to their toothbrush, but for the skin, called the Clarisonic. It costs over $200. I'm sure it's wonderful, but you can get pretty excellent results with a regular, $2 toothbrush.

When I began face brushing, in my 30s, I did it every couple of days. My skin built up a tolerance, and now, in my 40s, I do it at least once a day and sometimes twice. Start slowly and go easy. You have to test and see what your skin can tolerate. Obviously, you don't want to go overboard and brush the skin to the point of injury. You should not rub the skin off. I recommend a soft bristle brush. If, after a while, that doesn't feel like it's doing enough, you can move up to a medium bristle.

Brushing your skin regularly will improve its texture and tone and help soften lines and wrinkles. Always follow with a good moisturizer and be sure to apply sunscreen if you'll be outside.

TAKE OMEGA 3s

Part two of my mom's great combination is her advice to take Omega 3s every day, twice a day.

After a bit of research I found out that Omega 3s are highly recommend by the famed anti-aging doctor, author of *The Wrinkle Cure,* Doctor Nicholas Perricone. He touts a diet high in wild salmon, because of the fish's rich concentration of skin benefitting Omega 3s. And according to skin care expert Valerie Rosenbaum, studies have shown that supplementing with Omega 3s over a three month period improved skin firmness by 10%.

I had oily skin in my teens and 20s. In my mid-30s I noticed that the pores on some areas of my face were less oily and my skin was getting drier. Since I began taking the Omega 3 fish oil capsules, (two capsules of 1000mg or 1200mg twice a day) my skin is not dry and it looks more supple. The fine lines that were forming on my forehead and around my mouth have faded considerably.

For over a decade, I've been taking Omega 3 Fatty Acid capsules every day. As with all of the tips I'm sharing, "every day" is key. You must be consistent and make these things a habit if you wish to see results.

I recommend taking two Omega 3 capsules in the morning and two at night before bed.

The combination of the skin brushing, the Omega 3's, which I learned from mom, and protection from the sun (which I added myself) is what I most often share with women that ask why my skin looks so young. Those who do it and keep it up have great results. As I've said before, you must be consistent, though. The results come and last when you make the regimen a habit.

TAKE A MULTIVITAMIN EVERY DAY

I was in my thirties when I began to seriously consider why I was aging unusually slowly. At the time, I happened to have begun taking some new vitamins that I'd ordered through the mail. The company marketing the vitamins called and asked me to participate in a focus group it was conducting to track customers' response to the product.

At the session they asked me how long I had been taking vitamins. I realized I could not remember a time when I had *not* taken a multivitamin. Ever. I've taken vitamins from the time I could remember, since nursery school, at age 3. Back then my mother gave me sweet-tasting chewable children's vitamins and ever since I've taken a multivitamin just about every day of my entire life. It's always been a regular habit, like brushing my teeth. Though it would be hard to prove that this has contributed to why I've aged better than some, because it's just one among many anti-aging habits, I suspect that almost never having a vitamin deficiency cannot have hurt.

I read recently that Dr. Oz, (the popular guest on the Oprah Winfrey show who now has his *own* show), recommends a daily multivitamin as part of his anti-aging checklist. He advises breaking the vitamin in half, taking one part in the morning and the other at night. This, he says, ensures that the body has the right amount of fuel, as it needs it. According to Dr. Oz, if you take the entire vitamin at once, it's akin to over-filling your tank.

People have told me that vitamins and minerals are a waste of money, that we excrete most of them in our urine. Personal experience tells me otherwise. I've been anemic, taken iron tablets, and the anemia went away. I've had peri-menopausal discomfort, taken Vitamin B6, and the discomfort subsided. I've had cuts and scrapes, taken Vitamin C with bioflavonoids, and watched those wounds heal with amazing speed.

Vitamin A enhances the skin. Vitamin B2 enhances the growth of skin, hair and nails. B3 also enhances the health of skin. Vitamin C is an antioxidant and helps prevent skin damage. Vitamin E improves the skin by protecting fatty acids. It's also an antioxidant, so it has anti-aging benefits. Vitamin D enhances posture by protecting bones and muscles. Zinc also has antioxidant benefits that improve the skin.

I believe that taking these vitamins over the years is one of the things I've done consistently, in concert with other things, that has helped me maintain a youthful appearance well into my 40s.

Make taking a good multivitamin part of your daily routine.

EAT GELATIN

I discovered the benefits of eating unflavored gelatin accidentally. I was suffering from a painful shoulder condition and after reading that taking gelatin could be salutary for the joints, I began adding a packet a day to plain yogurt. After a few weeks of eating it regularly, I noticed that my skin looked better. The lines I had on the side of my mouth were less pronounced. After a few months, those lines were gone!

I began researching more about gelatin. It's made of animal collagen. Collagen is an essential protein. When you ingest it, it goes into you bloodstream and from there to your connective tissues, including your skin.

I recently saw a segment on Oprah.com about the anti-aging secrets of women in Japan. Instead of getting collagen injections, the women profiled in this story believed in eating collagen infused foods. The story showed them sneaking out of work to eat beef tendons. They were convinced that eating food high in animal collagen made their skin firmer. I don't doubt it. You'll be glad to know, however, that you can get the same results by adding unflavored gelatin to your diet. And what's even better is that unflavored gelatin is a mere 30 calories per pack and contains no fat or cholesterol.

According to a post on livestrong.com: "*A study published in a 2000 issue of the "Journal of New Remedies & Clinics," researchers studied the effect of collagen on the elastic properties of facial skin. The team found that taking a collagen drink that contains 5 g of collagen powder for five weeks significantly increased the flexibility of skin.*"

I recommend buying a 30-pack box of unflavored gelatin. It is sold in the baking goods section. Knox is a good brand, but you can also buy a store-brand version (it's the same stuff) that costs a few dollars less. When I began, I put in yogurt, but for the past few months I've been dissolving it in my morning drink. Empty the packet into a large cup. Add a bit of cold water, enough to cover the gelatin. Stir it until it dissolves. After that, add your hot liquid — coffee, tea, or whatever you drink, and stir. Consume as you normally would. You won't taste or notice the gelatin, as long as you drink it right away. If you leave it sitting, your coffee or tea may turn to jello.

When I published the first version of this book, gelatin was not included. I have had such excellent results, that I've updated the book to include it. If you take gelatin daily for just a few months, you will see such an improvement that you'll be a gelatin convert.

DRINK ALOE VERA JUICE

Aloe vera juice is great for the immune system and it's also beneficial for digestion throughout the entire digestive tract. According to Jeffery Bland, Ph.D who wrote the paper I mentioned previously: "Effect of Orally consumed Aloe Vera Juice," it has a tonic effect on the colon and it decreases bowel transit time. A well functioning colon will assist your body in maintaining skin that glows with youth and good health.

I began drinking the aloe vera juice to clear up acne, but I've continued to drink it a few times a week, even though my acne subsided long ago. I continue, because when I'm taking the juice, I notice that the quality of my skin is better. It's more vibrant and my pores appear to be cleaner and smaller. The whites of my eyes are brighter as well.

While suffering with adult acne I tried everything to control it. Retin-A made my skin red, raw and flakey. Antibiotics gave me a yeast infection. Accutane worked great while I was on it, but when I went off the medication, the acne returned.

I started drinking 8 ounces of pure aloe vera juice each day after a friend recommended it. Immediately I noticed that there were no more breakouts. Even during my pre-menstrual days, if I drank the juice faithfully no new pimples erupted. Everyone's body is different so some people may need more or less, but everyone I've told about it finds that it significantly improves their acne.

The taste of the pure juice can be unpleasant. Eventually I began mixing the juice with either fruit juice or lemonade and a little maple syrup and it still maintained its efficacy.

If you try it for acne control, once that is achieved you can reduce the amount you drink until you find what your body needs to keep your skin clear.

You might be inclined to skip over this information if you have no skin problems, but wait!

Even if you are acne free, I recommend Aloe Vera juice. It gently helps the colon move waste through the intestines. I think of it as a rinse for the colon, similar to what mouthwash does for the inside of your mouth. It doesn't have the extreme effect of a laxative, though, and so you can drink a glass a day without worrying that you'll need to remain close to a toilet.
Of course, everyone is different, so it's possible that its effect may be more pronounced on some than on others, but my experience has been that drinking it does not lead to the discomfort that laxatives can cause.

According to an article in *American Chronicle* aloe vera juice aids in weight loss by stimulating the metabolic rate in our liver cells so that we burn more energy. The article also claims that when you drink the juice, the body has to spend extra energy to assimilate its protein into the body and this extra energy expenditure also supports weight loss and muscle development. When I began to drink aloe vera juice I did find that maintaining my weight became less of an effort. I had thought it was because fewer calories may have been being absorbed from my food because of the slight laxative effect, but I see now that there's more to it than that.

Makers of aloe vera products claim that it reduces toxins and bacteria. I did a bit of research to see if I could find corroboration on this and it led me to the paper I mentioned by Jeffery Bland, Ph.D. According to Bland, after a controlled study wherein 10 subjects drank aloe vera juice and their stool was analyzed, the tests indeed found reduced bacteria in the colon as well as a reduction in fungal activity. My skin is clearer and brighter when I drink it and so I can believe it. I also feel greater vitality when I drink it. Both of these—clear, bright skin and vitality certainly contribute to a more youthful appearance.

Externally

You can reap the benefits of aloe vera by applying it to the body as well. For this, I recommend ALOE VERA GEL, in place of the juice. Look for a gel without added colors, fragrance or alcohol. Aloe vera is anti-bacterial, so applying it to the skin can reduce and even prevent breakouts. It's also very soothing and healing, so if your skin is irritated or inflamed, it can be helpful. It has astringent properties as well as being moisturizing, so it's great to use on the face for skin that is prone to breakouts, but also beginning to show signs of aging. It is said to be good for wrinkles, too.

APPLE CIDER VINEGAR

There are articles all over the Internet about the benefits of organic, non-pasteurized apple cider vinegar, which is said to have been used by Hippocrates as a heath tonic. This unpasteurized apple cider vinegar contains "the mother," a naturally occurring substance formed during the last step in fermentation. It has beneficial acids and enzymes that are removed in filtered apple cider vinegar.

Apple cider vinegar contains Malic Acid, which is thought to fight fungal and bacterial infections. The acid also dissolves uric acid deposits that form around the joints, which is believed to benefit those with arthritis. It is also known to reduce both blood glucose levels *and* the glycemic index of starchy foods. Unfortunately, many of these claims are thought to be mere folk remedies, and there are a number of articles refuting the claims.

In my experience, the vinegar *does* have health benefits, and I believe in its value as an anti-aging tool. For years I've been drinking a "tea" out of ACV, honey and water, though I drink less frequently now than I once did. I found its effects to be similar to those of aloe vera juice. It promotes regularity and it also helps keep my skin glowing. I suspect this is due to the antibacterial, detoxifying effect it is reported to have.

At times when I didn't have access to the aloe vera juice while I was combating acne, I was able to substitute a mixture of water, apple cider vinegar, and honey to keep my skin clear. For this reason, I believe it has a detoxifying effect on the body. I know that vinegar can be used as an antibacterial disinfectant externally, and that it's certainly safe to ingest, at least in moderation. And I can attest to the fact that since I began drinking the "tea" I've suffered far fewer seasonal colds than I did prior to taking it.

If you google the many articles on ACV, you'll find information on its benefits, and you'll also find articles debunking those claims. I can only tell you that I've tried it for many things, in addition to anti-aging, and I've had good results.

My recommendation is that you research it on your own. If it makes sense to you, give it a try—in moderation. I don't advocate drinking copious amounts, but try it in salad dressing, or make an occasional cup of the "tea."

Vinegar Tea:
2 tablespoons organic apple cider vinegar
1 cup hot water
1 tablespoon pure honey.

Combine all ingredients in a cup and stir.

A couple of caveats: The vinegar can have a deleterious effect on tooth enamel, so rinse your mouth after ingesting it. The other possible negative side effect is that it can adversely affect bone density if consumed regularly over long periods of time. So, don't drink it daily and don't overdo it. But I do recommend it as an addition to an anti-aging diet.

I've read countless testimonials on ACV and users repeatedly say they look much younger than their years. I know I do!

COCONUT OIL

Organic extra-virgin coconut oil is one of my favorite health and beauty products. It was first given to me by a beautiful and amazing woman in South Central Los Angeles. Her name is Anna Marie Carter, and she's the owner of a garden center in Watts, where she teaches people to grow food. She's known as "The Seed Lady." She offers instruction in organic gardening, and she shows people how to eat the way their elders did, consuming real foods grown in the earth. She is a goddess in my estimation.

I sought her out because of my interest in urban environmental issues. The day we met at her Watts Garden Center she treated me to a delicious lunch of broccoli, corn and mushrooms over brown rice that had been cooked with organic, extra-virgin coconut oil. It was fantastic, and I felt wonderful after eating it.

Internally

I began researching food grade coconut oil. I learned that the widely held belief that coconut oil is bad for us is actually false. It was believed that because it's a *saturated* fat, it contributed to heart disease, but this belief is changing. While it *is* a saturated fat, it is different from saturated animal fat, in that it does not contain cholesterol, and does not affect the body in the same negative way as animal fats do.

I ordered some on line and began cooking with the organic extra-virgin coconut oil three years ago. I read a book about the oil, called *The Coconut Oil Miracle*, which said that taken internally it promoted weight loss and added luster to the skin. I did not find the weight loss claim to be true for me. However, I did find that as I cooked my vegetables in it and added it to brown rice and sweet potatoes, my skin, indeed, appeared to have added luster. It seemed to lubricate the body inside and out.

Externally

Anna Marie Carter told me that coconut oil can be used not only for cooking, but also for the hair and body. This was corroborated in the book *The Coconut Oil Miracle.* As I mentioned, I've had acne prone skin, so I was nervous about putting the coconut oil on my face. It is, after all, *oil*, and oil usually clogs the pores. But I was in my early 40s when I tried it and though I was still prone to occasional adult acne, I was also curious about anything that combated aging. At first I limited its use to my forehead. Not only did it *not* break my skin out, it seemed to heal the remnants of a small blemish I had.

What I found out with further research was that coconut oil has anti-bacterial properties. Because it kills bacteria, it actually helps prevent acne. It can even be used under the arms in lieu of deodorant! This is because it kills the bacteria that causes odor. It can also be used as a massage oil and even as a sexual lubricant. Perhaps that's more information than you care to know-- but hey, good sex helps keep a body young, too!

Another wonderful benefit I found was that as my skin absorbed the oil, the tiny lines on my forehead, under my eyes, and around my mouth plumped up.

I now use it just about everyday on my face, entire body, and hair & scalp. In the morning, after washing (and scrubbing with the toothbrush), I put a thin layer of the oil on my face and neck and pat the excess off with a tissue. I apply a moisturizer with sunscreen on top of that.

I use it at night a few times a week, alternating with another oil (neem) that I'll discuss later. It is very hydrating. However, if your skin is particularly dry, you may need to re-apply it, because it is quickly absorbed. It's spectacular on dry feet, hands, elbows and knees as well. I use it all over the body after showering. I recommend applying it while the body is still damp.

Give it a minute, and then dry with a cotton towel or slip into a terry-cloth robe until dry. This will prevent the oil from getting on your clothes or sheets. If there is excess, towel it off with a cloth or paper towel.

Extra virgin, food grade coconut oil is a superb moisturizer and one that has no added chemicals or toxins. If you look at the ingredients of many body lotions, there are often lots of added chemicals. I try to limit the number of chemicals I put on my skin, as much as that's possible for me. (Though there are a few I cannot do without.) This is because it's difficult to discern what's toxic, and what isn't, and some toxins that we may put on our skin can be absorbed into the bloodstream. Except for sunscreen and a couple of other products, which I'll discuss later, I try not to use things on my skin that I could not safely eat. Coconut oil used in place of commercial body lotions, and in concert with other natural emollients, gives me the moisturizing I need to combat dry skin, without introducing unnecessary, undesirable toxins into my body.

I believe that chemicals that are not generally healthful, meaning they do nothing to nourish the body, are of no benefit. If they're not building the body up, they are likely breaking it down. Even if they are *not* breaking it down, if there is no tangible benefit to a chemical, I prefer to do without it.

By limiting unnecessary substances in body lotions and replacing them with ones that have health benefits, like those in coconut oil, and other natural ingredients, I feel I'm helping to reduce the toxins that, over time, contribute to aging.

Coconut oil is also excellent on the hair. I used it for a few months, applying at night and washing it out in the morning. I'd simply scoop some out with my fingers, rub in my hands to liquefy it, and then put it on my hair, from the scalp to the ends. After that, I'd put my hair in a bun and go to bed. If you want to try this, you might want to cover your hair with a scarf or bandana to protect your pillowcases, but it does wash out when you launder them. During that time, I was letting my hair dry naturally. One day I blew-dry it straight and I was stunned to see how shiny and healthy it was. It was in much better condition than the previous time I'd blown my hair dry and the only thing I had done differently was use the coconut oil. When I looked into this, trying to discover *why*, I found an article that claimed that coconut oil penetrates the hair shaft more effectively than other oils, which tend to merely *coat* the hair shaft. Coconut oil, according to what I read, gets deeper, resulting in a more lubricated strand of hair. It's been my experience that it conditions the hair better than any other product I've tried.

If you're at an age where you have to dye your hair because the gray is coming in, the peroxide in the dyes may be damaging your hair shaft. Conditioning with coconut oil will help. Well-conditioned, healthy hair contributes largely to a youthful appearance.

Pure, food grade coconut oil is a product that will benefit your body inside and out.

OLIVE OIL

Internally

It is widely known that consuming olive oil, which is rich in antioxidants, is beneficial for the heart, because it helps control bad cholesterol and raises the levels of good cholesterol. You should make it a habit to cook with olive oil, use it on salads, and enjoy it drizzled it over other foods. Olive oil deserves a place in any anti-aging regimen. And like fish oil and coconut oil, ingesting it will have a positive effect on your skin, helping to lubricate it from within.

In the 80s and 90s in my 20s and 30s, low-fat was all the rage. But a diet too low in fat leads to dry skin, hair and nails. A bit of the right fats in the diet, like fish oil, coconut oil and olive oil are great for your skin and will help keep it from wrinkling early. Your hair and nails need those fats to grow well, too, so do not be afraid to eat healthy fats in moderation. As we get older, we need them to look better, and when you're young if you make it a habit to incorporate them into your diet regularly you'll age better than if you did not.

Externally

Olive oil can be used on the hair similarly to the way I recommended using coconut oil. You can put it on at night, cover the hair with a scarf, and wash out in the morning. Or you can heat a couple of tablespoons in a small cup in the microwave, and use as a hot-oil treatment, washing it out right after, or the next day.

Some women use olive oil, with great success, on their skin. I tried this on my face and the result wasn't great for me—my skin responds better to coconut oil-- but, since my skin may be different from yours, I wouldn't rule out trying it if your skin is dry. Olive oil is high in antioxidants and vitamin E, so it does have the potential to soothe and heal.

I use it on my feet and find it excellent for keeping my heels well lubricated. Well-moisturized feet definitely look younger and prettier than dry, cracked, ashy feet!

I have also found that rubbing olive oil on my nails and cuticles nightly has been the best thing that's happened to them. Since I've entered my 40s, I've worked a lot more with my hands-- gardening, washing dishes, painting, sanding, cleaning. I bought a fixer upper house when I turned 40, and doing so much with my hands tends to destroy my nails. This is because I usually neglect to wear protective gloves, as I should. Being at the age of peri-menopause, when estrogen levels drop, also contributes to dryer nails. Gelatin capsules didn't work for me, unfortunately, but regular use of olive oil on my nails did wonders. It's great for the cuticles, too. And it doesn't hurt to rub it all over your hands and feet at night if you don't mind the smell.

NEEM OIL

My dear friend Apinya introduced me to neem oil when she gave me a bottle as a gift, along with a book on Ayurvedic beauty. Neem is a tropical Indian tree that has been used in Ayurvedic medicine.

Apinya told me that I could use the oil on my skin and scalp and that it was particularly beneficial for healing cuts, scratches, pimples, and insect bites. I first tried it on a couple of fleabites I'd gotten from a feral kitten who'd made her home in my backyard. Where I normally had an allergic reaction to insect bites that included swelling, the neem oil reduced the inflammation. Next I tried a few drops on some minor blemishes on my face, around my chin. The next day, those blemishes were barely noticeable.

I then began to search the Internet for more information on neem oil. I discovered that it has antibacterial properties and that there are many uses. As I searched, what most intrigued me was what I read about neem oil's effect on wrinkles. It is said to be an excellent moisturizer and one that works in the deeper layers of the skin.

One night, after brushing my face with the toothbrush as I've previously described, instead of following with the usual coconut oil, before I went to bed, I slathered some of the neem oil on the faint frown lines I have between my brows and I also put some on my laugh lines.

My skin liked the oil. It looked fantastic the next morning. The oil is, indeed, deeply penetrating. I don't favor the neem oil over the coconut oil, but I do like it very much and I recommend it. I use a combination of the coconut, and neem oil on my face, depending on what's going on with my skin.

It may seem like a bad idea to use any kind of oil if your skin is already oily. The neem oil, however, like coconut oil, is antibacterial. I've been using it with great results. It doesn't clog my pores or cause me to break out, even though I'm acne prone.

As we get older, those of us who suffer with acne may have the frustrating experience of having oily pores, even as our skin itself becomes drier and lines start to form. Neem oil is particularly good for women who are starting to get wrinkles *and* still suffer occasional breakouts.

What I didn't realize about neem oil that I feel compelled to share is that there are different kinds, and what you *really* need to know is that some smell better than others. "Pure" neem has a strong odor that may be off-putting to some people. I use a brand that primarily contains neem, and it is called neem oil, but it is actually alloyed with a few other oils, including sandalwood and Lavender that mitigate the smell.

SHEA BUTTER

I'm a relatively new user of Shea Butter. Shea and I got off to a rocky start. At first I was loath to recommend it, but as I've continued to give it a chance, it's grown on me and now I love it.

I had stumbled across the benefits of using Shea Butter as a moisturizer while researching other natural moisturizers. I read that it was great for lines and wrinkles and I wondered if it might be something I could use in combination with the neem oil and coconut oil to help combat fine lines.

I ordered some and when it came, the label said it was excellent on wrinkles. I put some on the fine lines on my forehead that I battle, continually. I decided to put some on the faint laugh lines I have as well. I slathered it on and went to bed.

When I woke up I had several pimples. My acne prone skin did not respond well to it at all. And those pimples took days to heal and left marks when they did. I was pretty ticked off at shea butter for a while. But then I began reading some forums on it on the web. I found one that said that it is, indeed, a great moisturizer, but not for the face of a person who is acne prone. True. However, an acne prone person can use it on other parts of the body and have wonderful results.

So I tried it again. I put it all over my feet one day, after a shower, and even at the end of the day, my feet were still soft and smooth. Then I tried it on my knees and elbows. Again, great results. I have since been using it everywhere but my face and my skin has responded very well to it.

Shea butter is thicker than the coconut oil, which absorbs into the skin. It sits on top of the skin and remains oily for a longer time. For extra-dry areas, this may work better than lighter ingredients, which disappear after a short time.

According to several articles I've read, shea butter contains vitamin's A and E, and something called cinnamic acid, all of which contribute to its anti-aging properties. A study conducted on cinnamic acid found that it could reduce melanin production, and so could be used for UV protection, and possibly as a skin lightener. I wouldn't recommend it in place of sunscreen, because it's not clear, exactly, how much protection it offers, but using it regularly on your skin could help reduce dark spots and other skin discolorations, giving you a more even-toned complexion, which certainly contributes to a more youthful appearance.

FASTING

I touched on fasting earlier and mentioned that when I was in my late 20s I was introduced to a fast called THE MASTER CLEANSE. The friend who turned me onto it, the actor, Tico Wells, is someone who has always looked about 20 years younger than his actual age and so I trusted that if it worked for him, it was definitely worth trying.

The Master Cleanse involves drinking laxative tea every day and drinking lemonade made out of fresh squeezed lemon juice, distilled water, grade B, pure maple syrup and cayenne pepper. There is also the saltwater flush, wherein one drinks a glass of water mixed with sea salt, which causes a bowel movement or two. Or three! On this fast all you consume is the tea, the lemonade, the salt water and all the distilled water you want.

I was supposed to do the fast for ten days, but didn't make the full ten. By the ninth day I was so desperate to chew something solid I began eating the lemons. And I began to drink the pure syrup from the bottle. It was time to quit. Even though I didn't complete the full ten days, I saw amazing benefits: Weight loss, glowing skin, and I felt happy and full of energy.

I sincerely felt like a new person physically and mentally. My thoughts were lighter and brighter. I felt like anything was possible and my energy was renewed, as was my enthusiasm for life.

They say that you actually clean out old waste, because the so-called "plaque" that forms on the walls of the colon over the years is broken down and washed out. But doctors that specialize in illnesses of the colon have dismissed the claims of "mucoid plaque" and if you view photos of the interior of the colon, you will see that there is nothing stuck to the walls of the organ.

The cells on the inside of the colon are similar to those inside the mouth and food doesn't remain stuck to it. However, I have empirical knowledge that when my colon was empty for a few days with nothing running through it but the Master Cleanse solution, the results were fantastic. While nothing *sticks* to the colon walls, having a clean colon and rinsing it out does have a positive effect on one's looks that is undeniable once you've experienced it.

What I believe, and what has worked for me, is that if you keep the body as pure as possible, and by this I mean free of unnecessary chemicals and unhealthful food additives, you will remain more youthful than if you continually expose yourself to unnatural, unhealthful substances. Cleansing removes unhealthful substances from the system, essentially allowing the body to start fresh; at least in theory.

Since doctors assert that the cleansing out of "old waste" is not, in fact, true, yet I still experienced visible benefits, I infer that these benefits may be due to something a little different from the cleansing of actual debris from the gastrointestinal walls. When I researched this, I read that the gastrointestinal wall can be separated into up to nine layers. So, it's possible that during the fast and the cleansing, toxins that pollute the body are drawn from the layers of tissue themselves, rather than from a layer of old fecal matter, as was originally claimed.

The Master Cleanse book claims that the laxative tea helps eliminate waste and the lemons and cayenne clean inside the colon. And according to the author, Stanley Burroughs, the combination of the maple syrup, lemons and cayenne have a good amount of vitamins and minerals. I certainly had enough energy and it felt exhilarating to be so clean inside.

If there are accumulated toxins in your body as a result of a poor diet, it makes sense that it would be aging, and that if you clean it out your body will feel "new," in a sense. Ideally our bodies function well enough to remove toxins naturally through our liver, kidneys and the skin, but when we're repeatedly exposed to chemical additives perhaps the body's ability to detox gets sluggish. When you focus on cleansing periodically, you accelerate the process and you really do feel the difference.

I have never been able to do the fast again for more than 3 days, but 3 days seems to be enough for me. Despite naysayers who claim *The Master Cleanse,* does nothing but cause one to lose weight because of caloric reduction, I recommend it, albeit with some caveats. You can find it in New Age book stores and online. If you plan on doing it for the full 10 days I would recommend being under the care of a physician or holistic doctor to be safe. If you can only do it for 3 to 5 days, that will have some positive effects, too. Take care to break the fast gradually, beginning with soup and vegetable salads. **And please, if you're diabetic or have some other health issue that might make the ingredients in the fast dangerous for you, don't try it.**

The other type of fasting that is beneficial and youth enhancing is fresh juice fasting. I recommend a juice fast once every few weeks, where you begin at 5pm and drink nothing but fresh juices, water and aloe vera juice until 5 pm the next day. Thereafter you can break the fast with some vegetable soup or a salad and resume normal eating the following day.

I recommend fresh carrot, parsley, beet, spinach and celery in any combination. You can add lemon or ginger. It's best if you can buy a juicer and make the juices yourself, but if not you can use juices from the health food store if they're fresh. Too much carrot juice can briefly turn your skin orange, so don't go crazy with it. Drink a lot of water and herbal tea if you have to, but nothing else but the juice. No coffee or soda. This is not a fast to lose weight, though you might lose a pound or two. The point of the juice fast is to cleanse, give your digestive system a mini rest and to give your body something really healthy to nourish it. You will feel and look great after juicing for a day. It may inspire you to eat more healthfully thereafter.

DRINK ONLY LIQUIDS THAT HAVE NUTRITIONAL VALUE, CLEANSE, OR HYDRATE

If it does nothing GOOD for your body, you don't need it.

I stopped drinking sodas and diet sodas in the early 90s. Diet soda is not a healthful or youth enhancing drink, though diet soda may help some people keep their weight down.

There are better choices that can be made for a calorie free or low calorie drink. I was actually heavier when I was drinking diet sodas. When you begin to eat healthfully, only putting things into your body that nourish it, hopefully you will eliminate diet soda. If you want a calorie free drink you are much better off drinking water or unsweetened green tea or even black coffee.

Look at the ingredients listed on a can of soda either diet or regular. They're full of chemicals! Some may be harmless, but some are not. For example, phosphorus, one of the chemicals found in sodas, can contribute to osteoporosis, because it depletes the bones of calcium. If you cut out soda as soon as possible, your bones have a better chance of staying strong as you age.

Going back to my theory that keeping our bodies as free of toxins as possible will have a youth enhancing effect, the chemical additives in sodas have no place in a diet that aims to reduce toxins. Think of it this way, whatever we ingest becomes part of us; it enters our bloodstream and the cells of our body. Why would you want your cells to be bathed in the chemical ingredients of soda, alcohol, or sugary drinks?

If it's not building you up, it's probably breaking you down.

If you want to assist your body in staying healthy and youthful, please avoid ingesting liquids that have no benefit to your body.

Drink water. You can drink it all day long and it's great for you. It hydrates your skin, helps flush out toxins and even magically seems to melt fat off. If you begin to drink eight, 8oz glasses a day, you will see an improvement in the quality of your skin and you will probably eat slightly less. Try drinking water with some lemon or lime squeezed into it if water alone is too boring. Or make your own healthy lemonade with water, lemons and maple syrup or honey.

And if you drink juice, drink *real* juice, not "juice drinks" with added sugar or high fructose corn syrup. Look at the labels and choose products that are 100% pure juice. "From concentrate" is okay, as long as it doesn't contain added sweeteners. Avoid sugar, high fructose corn syrup, and "diet" sweeteners.

Too much coffee is not great for youth either, but a cup or two a day is actually good. (Just don't add white sugar or artificial sugar substitutes.)

Recently there's been evidence to suggest that coffee is very high in antioxidants. This is excellent news for coffee drinkers like me! Antioxidants are substances in foods that can prevent or slow the oxidative damage that free radicals cause to our bodies. Free radicals occur when our body cells use oxygen and they can cause damage that leads to health problems.

If, like me, you *must* drink coffee, I completely understand, but too much caffeine can affect your heart rate and contribute to stress. It can also raise cholesterol levels and lead to insomnia. All of these can be aging. It was believed that caffeine was dehydrating as well, though more recent studies dispute this. However, I *can* see the difference in my skin when I drink two cups of coffee in the morning and nothing else by noon, as opposed to when I drink one cup of coffee and a couple of glasses of water. Less coffee + more water = better looking skin.

If you want to develop habits that over time are going to help you stay younger looking, my advice is to limit your coffee/caffeine intake to one or two 8oz cups a day, at most.

Caffeine can have a terrible effect on one's ability sleep so refrain from ingesting it late in the day. Poor sleep, over time, will accelerate the aging process.

Doctors recommend that we drink some red wine a few times a week. I don't recommend drinking alcohol or anything that has no nutritional value, except for red wine, and only in moderation. Red wine contains antioxidants and it's beneficial to the heart. Lately there's been a lot of discussion about the antioxidant found in red wine called Resveratrol.

In an article published by the Mayo Clinic, research has shown that, Resveratrol can actually reverse the signs of aging. I've been hearing about the heart benefits it offers for a while now, but just recently I read an article that claimed the Resveratrol you'd get from drinking a glass of red wine each day also improves bone density. Good bone density is a key component to staying young looking. The heart benefits of red wine are realized because the antioxidants help prevent blood clotting and they also relax blood vessels, inhibiting the oxidation of bad cholesterol.

In general, alcohol is dehydrating and bad for your organs. It's a diuretic and flushes water from the body. This robs your skin of nutrients and moisture that are vital to cellular function. Dehydrated skin looks older.

Alcohol, due to its diuretic effect, causes your kidneys to work harder as they remove water from your system. Too much alcohol can permanently damage the liver. The liver breaks down alcohol so it can be removed from the body. If more alcohol is consumed than the liver can remove, this creates an imbalance that can harm the liver because the overload interferes with its breakdown of fats, proteins and carbohydrates.

So, if looking and staying youthful is your goal, don't be a heavy drinker. You want to do things to keep your organs healthy. Harming them is certainly not going to benefit your overall health and it's definitely not going to help you look better or younger. Drinking in moderation is okay, but consistent drinking over the years will contribute to aging you faster than if you limit your alcohol intake.

Green tea is a good choice to add to the list of healthful drinks. It has been shown to reduce cholesterol. It's also said to be an aid in weight-loss. And it is rich in the antioxidant epigallocatechin gallate (EGCG) which is said to kill cancer cells without harming healthy tissue.

According to the well-known anti-aging specialist, Dr. Nicholas Perricone, author of *The Wrinke Cure,* green tea is a better morning drink than coffee, because green tea does not cause a spike in cortisol levels the way too much coffee can. Cortisol is an adrenal steroid that is believed to be an age accelerator. Perricone even asserts that replacing green tea for coffee will result in weight loss due to the reduction in cortisol production. For me, life just isn't as sweet without my morning cup of coffee, but I have made green tea a part of my diet because of all the health and anti-aging benefits and I recommend that you make it part of yours as well.

Avoid beverages with added sugar. This includes some flavored waters and sports drinks. Sugar is aging. According to an article, "Sugar Speeds up the Aging Process," by Jennifer Guevin, a study in the British Journal of Dermatology found that eating sugar contributes to developing wrinkles. Guevin's article states:

"When glucose enters the bloodstream, it latches onto proteins in the body. As it turns out, collagen and elastin, the proteins that help keep skin elastic, are two of the most susceptible proteins to this process, according to the study."

Avoid "diet" sweeteners as well. They are full of chemicals that do nothing to promote good health and are more than likely harmful. Avoid them both. Sparingly use honey, molasses, or maple syrup in place of refined white sugar. You may have heard of Agave syrup, which is another alternative. There's some controversy around Agave, however, and I'm not convinced of its health benefits.

You can use honey, molasses or maple syrup to sweeten coffee, tea or other drinks. Honey may a form of sugar and not be a super health food, but it does have *some* nutritional benefits (vitamins and minerals) and it's an antioxidant. Maple syrup *does* have significant nutritional benefits. It contains calcium, potassium and iron. Molasses contains calcium, potassium, magnesium and is a good source of iron. I've had people balk at the idea of sweetening coffee with honey, molasses or maple syrup, but it's actually good and any one of them is better for you than white sugar.

EAT ONLY (OR AT LEAST MOSTLY) FOODS THAT HAVE NUTRITIONAL VALUE

Okay, this may be impossible to do ALL the time. Part of any good plan for staying youthful certainly includes enjoying life (!) so I'm not saying you can *never* eat a special treat *on occasion*. I do. But, habitually, I make it a point to eat foods that I know are doing something beneficial for my body. I don't eat empty calorie foods most of the time and neither should you. By these I mean junk food—candy, cake, donuts, chips, artificially colored and flavored foods or drinks, soda, etc.

Think of eating as something you do to look and feel great. Love your body enough to fill it with WHOLE FOODS that are nourishing, and your body will reflect that. You really *are* what you eat.

By "whole foods," I mean those that are unprocessed, or processed and refined as little possible before we eat them. Whole foods contain no additives. They are what they are: a piece of fruit, a vegetable, whole grains, beans, nuts, seeds, eggs, fresh fish, you get the idea. These foods are grown or raised. They are *real*. Whole foods do not contain a list of chemical additives. They are foods in their most natural state.

I learned to eat properly back in the early 90s when I realized I was twenty pounds overweight. I was was living in New York City, walking everywhere and working out at the McBurney YMCA, doing cardio and lifting weights, but my diet was terrible. I would overeat things that I thought were healthy, like frozen yogurt and items from the salad bar at the deli. I drank gallons of diet soda, ate tubs of so-called "diet butter," went through boxes of Equal and artificial creamer in my coffee, chewed several packs of sugar-free gum a day, and ate snacks from the health food store constantly, thinking that "healthy" meant that the calories didn't count.

One day I woke up, weighed myself and I was over 140 pounds. At 5'4" it didn't look good on me. I was pursuing an acting career at the time and was being sent up for ingénue roles, but at that weight, I didn't have an ingénue body. As I got off and on the scale again, in tears, re-checking the number that kept coming up, hoping the thing was broken, I remembered my friend Claudia, whom I'd met in an acting class, telling me that she'd learned how to eat properly by doing Weight Watchers. She looked great and had stayed slim consistently. I signed up later that day.

Weight Watchers taught me a balanced way of eating, one that allows all types of foods in a combination that makes the metabolism work most efficiently. You can eat carbohydrates, protein, even fat. In my estimation this makes more sense than diets that completely eliminate certain food groups, because those diets feel more like a *diet*, whereas the Weight Watchers plan is a way of eating that can be maintained for life.

I recommend eating a protein, vegetables and/or fruit at each meal. Add some sort of whole grain product to one or two meals such as brown rice, oatmeal or whole wheat bread. I recommend whole grains over breads or pasta, because whole grains are "whole food," and better for the body than white breads or white pastas, but I realize not everyone can give up bread entirely. So, if that's you, at least opt for high fiber whole grain varieties over white bread. Carbohydrates that are lower in fiber have a higher glycemic index and the body converts them to glucose quickly, which means that they cause rapid spikes in blood sugar. The body digests whole grains more slowly. These foods cause a slower change in blood sugar, which is more desirable.

For calcium, add some low-fat dairy, (my recommendation is plain, unsweetened yogurt with active cultures) or soy if you're vegan and have found your body tolerates soy products. (Keep in mind that soy contains estrogen and too much of it can cause problems in some people. Try to limit soy intake to one or two servings per day.)

Include nuts in the diet, almonds and walnuts especially. Too many nuts can cause weight gain, but in moderation they're healthful. They provide fiber and protein and they help prevent heart disease.

Limit the fat, but don't omit it entirely. Use olive oil or coconut oil for cooking. Avoid deep fried foods. Use skinless chicken and lean meats. Avoid processed meats like bacon, salami or pepperoni.

With fish, chicken and meats, try to eat them as close to their pure state as possible. By pure state I don't mean raw, except for sushi and sashimi, which I do recommend. What I mean by "close to their pure state," is without additives or extras. For example, a piece of chicken or fish grilled, or sautéed in olive oil, chopped garlic and spices is a an example of the fish or chicken prepared in a way that is close to it's natural state. A piece of fish or chicken dipped in batter, stuffed with breadcrumbs and deep fried is not. A broiled piece of steak is a whole food. A hot dog, salami, or sausage, which is processed meat, is not.

Brown rice, oatmeal, and other whole grains are a better choice than processed cereals, breads and pastas. There is nothing added to brown rice or unsweetened oatmeal. Whole grains are whole foods; they are what they are and you can control what you put in them, so you know they are fully nutritious.

When you eat highly nutritious foods, you can't help but vibrate better health (and youth) than when you eat processed, lower quality food. When you continually nourish your body with high quality food, year after year, you are going to age much more slowly than if you feed your body low quality food. So eat better, if you want to look better.

RAW FOODS

If you really want to glow and look vibrant and youthful, incorporate several raw foods into your diet each day.

In the late 90s I was in Chicago visiting my sister one winter and discovered a raw food restaurant there. It was my first time seeing one. The owner was a gorgeous woman in her 50s who could have passed for someone in her 30s. She was slim, radiant, and absolutely stunning.   She inspired me.

After seeing how magnificent this woman looked I decided to research the raw food diet and I gave it a try. I found that a *completely* raw food diet, year round, is not for me. I developed anemia and became deficient in vitamin B12. However, short periods of eating "raw only" works well for me. And incorporating a ratio of about 60% raw to 40% cooked food, daily, works for me. The percentages are just a guess, but I think a good one.

Everyday, I'm sure to eat a few pieces of raw fruit, a salad or two with several raw vegetables, and some raw nuts. Raw foods are clean foods, high in fiber. The high fiber content helps to keep the digestive system healthy. Many raw foods also have a high water content and are low in calories (except nuts and seeds), which help in shedding excess weight. Eat more of them and you will be more regular, feel lighter, leaner, and look younger.

To do a completely raw food diet will require a lot of research. Though it's not for me, I do recommend it if it's something that interests you. Just about everyone I've met who eats totally raw looks youthful and amazing. But if you cannot or don't want to do an exclusively raw diet, definitely eat several raw foods each day, every day. Raw food has vibrancy and energy and when you see someone who eats plenty of raw fruits, vegetables and nuts you can actually see and feel that energy radiating from them. This may sound like nonsense to skeptics and if it does to you, I can understand that. But consider that everything is made up of energy. The energy in raw foods is vibrant with life. A diet rich with that vibration—the colors, the moisture, the nutrients, can't help but translate into a body that thrives with vitality.

EAT A VARIETY OF COLORS

This will be easy if you eat fruits and vegetables, which you should be doing if you're looking to vibrate youth! The colors in fruits and vegetables are energizing and revitalizing. They benefit us psychologically because they're vibrant, beautiful and alive. They benefit us physiologically, because they're full of nutrients. I get such a boost from eating a fruit salad filled with blueberries, raspberries, bananas, pineapple and kiwi, or a salad with spinach, tomatoes, corn, and red onion. The variety of colors just feels so wonderful to me. And it really is! Eating a rainbow assortment of fruits and veggies is a great way to nourish your body with what it needs to strengthen your immune system, detoxify, and combat the aging process.

Different colors benefit in different ways.

For example, many **yellow and orange** foods contain vitamin A and carotenes, like carrots, yams, yellow squash, cantaloupes, mangoes. These are great for the eyes, skin and they reduce cancer risk and help the immune system.

Other orange foods like citrus fruits don't contain vitamin A, but they do contain Vitamin C and folate. (Folate helps create new body cells which is why it is recommended that pregnant women take it.)

Anthocyanins, powerful antioxidants that protects cells from damage, are found in **blue and purple** foods like blueberries, blackberries, grapes eggplant and raisins.

Red fruits and vegetables contain lycopene and anthocyanins. Lycopene helps reduce the risk of cancer. And as stated above, anthocyanins are antioxidants that prevent cell damage. Lycopene is found in cooked tomatoes. Anthocyanins are found in strawberries, red grapes and raspberries.

Green fruits and vegetables contain lutein, which helps the eyes. They also contain folate, which prevents birth defects. And they contain nutrients that help protect against cancer. The green foods include: spinach, broccoli, kiwi, zucchini, green beans, green apples and cabbage.

Some **White** fruits and vegetables contain the healthy compound allicin, which contains antibacterial and anti fungal properties. Garlic is high in allicin, which is also said to lower cholesterol and reduce the risk of heart disease. Other white foods like potatoes and bananas are good sources of potassium.

Using color in the diet doesn't have to stop with fruits and vegetables, though. Keeping color in mind can help you vary your diet in other ways. Try to get reds, whites, greens, blues, yellows, oranges and even pinks, blacks, browns and beiges in the diet.

Consider salmon and shrimp for the pinks. Consider nuts, oatmeal, brown rice and lentils or beans for the beiges. For blacks and browns, try prunes, black beans, figs or dark chocolate (which contains healthful antioxidants) and even cooked lean meat.

Here's a list of the things I eat/drink regularly: coffee, almond milk, low-fat regular (cow's) milk, unsweetened cocoa, blueberries, oatmeal, walnuts, almonds, oranges, apples, cantaloupe, honey, green tea, grape juice, carrot juice, maple syrup, eggs, non-fat or low-fat plain yogurt, broccoli, spinach, salmon, tuna, chicken, leafy salad greens, tomatoes, corn, green peas, red onions, apple cider vinegar, olive oil, coconut oil, brown rice, quinoa, black beans, beets, carrots, carrot juice, red peppers, sweet potatoes, dark chocolate, and red wine.

I also eat things that aren't on this list, but not all the time. Many of the items on the list are considered "super foods," that are healthful and beautifying. Try to incorporate some of them into your diet.

AVOID TOO MUCH ALCOHOL

I know drinking is fun, but there is so little nutritional value in liquor that it's a waste of calories. However, as I mentioned earlier, there are several health benefits to drinking some red wine a day. If you must drink, I would recommend that you stick with red wine in moderate amounts.

Other types of alcohol in moderation, on occasion, won't completely ruin your ability to age well. Who can resist a class of champagne or a cold beer once in a while? But too much drinking will not *help,* if your objective is to stay young looking.

I came from a household where alcohol was always available. I drank as a teenager in high school, and also in college. Social drinking seemed inevitable. But even then I could see that I did not look well on the days after drinking a lot.

My vanity kicked in fairly early in life, and since my early 20s, I've limited my drinking to a couple of glasses of wine at time.

I went to a reunion recently and the looks of the people who admitted to being heavy drinkers had suffered. Those who were heavy drinkers *and* heavy smokers had fared even worse. I didn't recognize several of them. Their faces and bodies appeared swollen. Their skin looked dull. Their voices had gotten deep and raspy, and the way they carried themselves suggested sluggishness and ill health. It wasn't until I saw photos posted on the Internet that I realized who some of them were. And these were people I'd known from kindergarten, through high school! They had aged beyond recognition.

Too much alcohol damages neural connections in the brain and dehydrates your body. Your liver, stomach, kidneys and pancreas are also adversely affected. In a lifestyle dedicated to staying healthy and youthful, sustained alcohol consumption has no place. Cut back or cut it out.

NOOOOOO SMOKING!

Obviously you don't need me to tell you not to smoke. Smoking is *terrible* for your health and is very aging. Anything that wreaks havoc on any of your organs is going to age you. Do not smoke, ever, if you are looking to maintain a youthful appearance. There are no exceptions to this! Even occasional smoking is harmful.

Smoking is not only aging, but it causes numerous health problems, bad breath, yellow teeth and wrinkles. It's also selfish to do in public, because second-hand smoke is harmful and uncomfortable to others.

If you are in your 20s or 30s and you smoke, QUIT NOW! If you don't smoke, please don't ever start. You will age so much more gracefully without smoking.

Think of the women you know. Do you know any heavy smokers age 50 or older? How about non-smokers 50 or older? Is there a difference in the appearance in the skin and bodies of these women? How about the quality of their voices? I bet there is.

AVOID TOO MANY PLASTIC CONTAINERS

The information accessible regarding plastic containers is conflicting and confusing. There are articles online that claim that there are dioxins in plastic water bottles and that if you put them in the freezer or allow them to sit in a hot car in the sun, the dioxins seep into the liquid contained in the bottle. According to an interview with a researcher at Johns Hopkins University, Dr. Rolf Halden, this is a myth. He says that plastics do not contain dioxins.

However, chemicals found in another type of plastic container, the heavier plastic intended for multiple use, are said to be one of the main sources of synthetic oestrogens in the body. Oestrogens trigger fat deposition and this is worsened if you're also exposed to syntheic oestrogens in the environment. Bisphenol A is one of the chemicals that I've read is contained in some plastic water bottles and is transferred from the plastic into liquids. Bisphenol A is thought to be linked to several types of cancer.

The best thing to do is research this on your own, compare the articles and decide for yourself. I tend to favor being safe rather than sorry, so I'm currently using a metal canteen to carry my water.

If there is a possibility that something contains harmful chemicals and I can choose an alternative, I prefer to do that. As I've said over and over, I believe that toxins contribute to the aging process.

I'd also like to encourage you to avoid microwaving food in plastic containers when possible. Studies suggest that Bisphenol A leaches into the food heated in plastic containers. One study claims that the amounts detected were high enough to cause neurological and developmental damage in laboratory animals. To be safe, please transfer food into ceramic or glass containers when you microwave.

Any amount of chemicals or toxins that find their way into what I'm drinking or eating disturbs me. Think about eating the way people did years ago. Plastics weren't as ubiquitous as they are now. People used glass bottles rather than plastic. They cooked in real ovens and on stoves, and ate fewer processed foods.

Any opportunity you can take to eat and drink food or liquid that has *not* been exposed to toxins is going to be beneficial. Make this a habit and over time, limited exposure to these toxins will benefit your looks as well as your health.

REMOVE YOUR MAKEUP AND WASH AND MOISTURIZE YOUR FACE EVERY NIGHT

This is a life-long habit every woman should cultivate without exception. Do not go to sleep without removing your makeup, washing and moisturizing. If you make this an unbreakable habit you will train yourself to care for your skin consistently. Being consistent is one of the most important keys to any beauty regimen. You must do things regularly in order to have lasting, cumulative benefits.

If you keep up the habit of never going to bed without removing your makeup, washing your face and moisturizing not only will your skin thrive and be healthy, but you will be able to incorporate additional beauty aids, such as the skin brushing, taking the Omega 3s and the tooth brushing and flossing. Cultivating everyday dedication to your own upkeep will serve you very well, because you'll be more likely to make all the elements of your health and beauty routine habitual.

If you skip days of washing your face at night, you are more likely to skip eating properly, exercising and everything else you do, routinely, to maintain your looks.

Skin can become dehydrated at night, especially in the winter months when you turn the heat up. This takes moisture out of the air and your skin needs extra hydration, so moisturizing at night is essential.

One of the best tips I've come across recently was one I saw in a beauty magazine at the nail salon. The advice had come from the writer's mother, who had recommended that she keep her moisturizer near the toilet at night, so when she got up to go to the bathroom, she could apply it again. This would give her the opportunity for three applications: morning, night and middle of the night, instead of just two. I have tried to do this as often as I can and think it's a wonderful idea. Wish I'd thought of it!

During sleep your body repairs muscles and tissues, including skin, as dead or aging cells are replaced. Cleansing your skin at night before sleep will assist the restorative process, making it easier for the body to repair or replace your skin cells, as it doesn't have the disruption of a layer of makeup, dirt or extra bacteria. And if you use a night cream formulated specifically to work during sleep, you can reap added benefits.

If you're in your 20s or 30s begin to make nightly makeup removal, washing, and moisturizing a life-long habit. Over time, this will result in keeping your skin in good shape. If you're older and you don't cleanse your skin regularly at night, start now. It's not too late to cultivate this as a new habit. As you cleanse and moisturize regularly, pampering your older skin, you will slowly begin to see results of added luster and reduced fine lines and this will inspire you to continue. And as you pamper your maturing skin regularly, this will even build self-esteem, because caring for your skin is an act of self-love. As you love and care for yourself, regularly nurturing your skin in this way, you cannot avoid looking and feeling better and more youthful.

WIDE BRIMMED HATS AND SUNSCREEN

When I was 33, I had an appointment with my dermatologist, because I was still combating acne. While I was sitting in the waiting room, I read an article written by another dermatologist, who said that she never went outside without a wide brimmed hat and sunscreen.

I thought of my mother, who has aged wonderfully and I recall that she never, ever wanted to sit out in the sun without a hat. I used to tease her for not wanting to get darker. She came up in a time and place where if you were black, which she is, the culture dictated that the lighter your skin, the better off you were. But that wasn't all there was to her decision to avoid too much sun. She knew that sun exposure contributed to premature aging.

The woman who'd written the article was Caucasian, very fair, with blond hair, and said she was 60. From what I could tell in the photos, her skin looked decades younger. Skin with less melanin tends to show its age earlier than darker skins, and hers was very light. Yet, she looked incredibly youthful.

She stressed repeatedly that protecting the skin from the sun was the *single, most important thing people could do to prevent aging.* Please make a note of this, because sun protection cannot be stressed enough if you are interested in remaining youthful-looking for as long as possible.

She recommended looking at the skin on one's buttocks, which, presumably, has been covered when outdoors, and comparing it to the skin on the hands or face. Of course the skin that's been covered looks much more supple than the exposed skin. Granted, the tissue under the skin of the hands is far thinner than tissue of the buttocks, which accounts for some of the difference in the way these areas age, but her point is still well taken.

That was the day I decided to become even more diligent about wearing hats. In my 20s, while living in New York City, I wore hats constantly, just because I loved them. It was about fashion. This was fortuitous, because wearing them all that time reduced my sun exposure, which contributed to my aging well.

When I moved to LA, at first, I worshipped the sun a little too much. I bought a convertible and found I received more compliments when I had a tan. I, too, believed I looked better with some color. This may have been true in the short term, but I eventually realized that my long-term goal of staying young looking was more important than having that bronzed look. Besides, you can always apply bronzer or self-tanner.

After reading that article in the dermatologist's office I thought back to the very first time I'd noticed lines on my young skin at age 15. I'd spent 3 weeks on vacation baking on the beach in Barbados with no sunscreen. At that age, and at that time (in the 70s) I wasn't cognizant of the damage I could be causing, and even if someone had told me about it, I was so young I felt invincible.

When I returned to the states and was going into 10th grade, one morning I noticed lines on my forehead while looking in the mirror, getting ready for school. I knew that they were the result of the very dark tan I'd gotten, but I didn't worry too much about it. But now, when I read about how most aging has to do with sun exposure, I know from experience that it's true. If the sun could put lines on my young, healthy, 15-year-old face, then clearly it will wreak havoc on a face twice or three times that age.

Now, I almost never go outside without a hat in the daytime. This has been a strict habit since that day in the doctor's office, in my early 30s. Though I don't always wear a wide-brimmed hat, I try to when it works with what I'm wearing. Usually I'm dressed in workout gear, and so I'll wear a ball cap. If you can wear a wide-brimmed hat most of the time, I'd recommend that, since it will shade your entire face and neck, whereas the ball cap leaves some areas exposed.

I also wear sunscreen everyday if I'm going outside. I use SPF 30 or higher. I started wearing sunscreen in my moisturizer when I was 24. If you're in your 20s, start wearing it now. In fact, I don't think people are ever too young to begin wearing sunscreen daily. Even if it's not sunny outside there are UV rays.

Hands

Don't forget to put sunscreen on your hands! Hands are one of the first areas of the body to show their age. Too much sun exposure leads to age spots and dried out wrinkled hands. Begin wearing sunscreen on your hands early in life, because they are constantly exposed to the sun. My hands look pretty good, but they'd probably look better had I begun wearing sunscreen on them in my 20s. I didn't begin paying attention to them until my 30s.

If your hands look old and sun damaged try exfoliating them regularly with a scrub or a loofah and hydrating them nightly with olive or coconut oil.

Vitamin D

And now for some confusing and contradictory information: What I've advised could cause you to suffer a lack of Vitamin D! Human skin produces Vitamin D as a result of being exposed to the sun. Our bodies need this vitamin and many of us are deficient in it, because we don't spend enough time in the sun during the summer months or if we do, we're covered up, or slathered with sunscreen. Using sunscreen prohibits the skin's ability to make vitamin D when it's exposed to the sun. Among the diseases associated with lack of Vitamin D are: osteoporosis, heart disease, and breast, colon and prostate cancer. So, what is a person interested in aging well supposed to do? Get some sun in the spring and summer, but be wise about it. Do protect your face and hands as I've suggested. But several days a week or at least on the weekends, try to expose your arms, legs, back or stomach to the sun for 15 minutes at a time without sunscreen. Be sure to moisturize this skin daily. And consider eating plenty of tomatoes and red peppers. They contain lycopene which helps the skin tolerate sun with less damage.

BRUSHING, FLOSSING, PEROXIDE

Brushing one's teeth twice daily is a must. You don't need me to tell you that, you've heard it for years. Still, I am surprised by the number of people I know who don't brush at least twice a day. Having white teeth takes years off your appearance. If you brush after drinking coffee or red wine, you can prevent staining. And brushing regularly and seeing a dentist once or twice a year will help prevent periodontal disease. Periodontal disease can lead to other health problems including heart disease and diabetes.

Brush your tongue, too. The back of the tongue can build up bacteria that cause bad breath. Some bacteria in the mouth are beneficial, but when they multiply and smell, bacteria are not doing you or your body any good.

Floss Once a Day

I once heard a study that said flossing the teeth daily has an anti-aging effect on the body. I didn't understand why that would be so, but back in the mid 90s a dental hygienist encouraged me to floss daily since that would prevent plaque from building up. She explained that it takes 24 hours for plaque to calcify, so flossing at least once a day would prevent tartar build up. Mostly due to vanity, I have been flossing daily since then.

Not long ago, I came across an interview with internist Michael Roizen author of *REAL AGE: Are You as Young as You Can Be?* He said that the bacteria in plaque that cause periodontal disease set up an immune reaction that causes inflammation in your arteries. This, according to Roizen, can lead to aging of your arteries, heart disease, stroke, memory loss, impotence and-- wrinkling of your skin! Surprised? I was. But good to know! Floss at least once a day every day!

Peroxide

Forgive me. I hate how this is going to sound, but it's true. I have, hands down, the whitest teeth of anyone I know. For most of my life dentists have told me that my teeth are among the whitest of their patients.

One of my dentists actually said:

"When I see a mouth like yours, I have mixed emotions. I'm happy to see teeth so well cared for, but if all my patients were like you, I'd be out of business."

I have never used whitening strips, nor have I had my teeth professionally bleached. My secret? Since the age of 12, I've used store bought peroxide as a dental rinse. Yes, that's my inexpensive (50-cent) secret. It was at that time that my father showed me how he mixed peroxide and baking soda and brushed his teeth with it. I didn't feel like doing that. Call me crazy, but I just preferred toothpaste.

However one day, my teeth felt particularly dirty and sticky from candy and I figured if you can mix peroxide and baking soda, you can probably just use the peroxide as a mouthwash.

I poured a bit into my mouth, swished it around, and let it sit for a few seconds. My gums felt weird—they tingled and I spit the peroxide out, careful not to swallow any. My gums had turned white in a few places and even looked like they'd kind of been eaten away! It terrified me! But soon, they went back to their normal pink. All was well, to my great relief.

I tried it again the next day and my gums didn't turn white, they were fine. I deduced that there had been something in my gums that needed some sterilizing or at least some attention, and the peroxide had healed them. From then on, every few days, I would pour a little peroxide in my mouth and let it do its thing.

Eventually I learned that peroxide *is*, in fact, a dental rinse. It is recommended that you dilute it with water before using it, though! If you don't dilute it, your teeth will likely become over sensitive. I've been rinsing my teeth with straight peroxide a few times a week for more than 30 years, and though my teeth are pearly white, and my dentist assures me my enamel is fine, my teeth are *very* sensitive to cold foods. I have a friend who's dentist and she doesn't recommend that people ever rinse with straight peroxide. Follow the directions on the bottle and mix with an equal amount of water. Swish in the mouth for one minute and then spit out. According the directions you can do this up to 4 times per day, after meals and at bedtime. Do this and your teeth will sparkle. Your gums will be healthy, too!

A friend who had never used peroxide and thought it sounded weird began to rinse his teeth with it a few times a week about a year ago and his teeth are almost as white as mine now.

White teeth definitely help you look younger. But you don't need to do expensive professional bleaching or even use bleaching strips to get them. An average bottle of peroxide costs under a dollar!

WALK, WALK, WALK, WEIGHTS, WATER

I learned anti-aging and beauty tips from my mother, but it was my father who taught me the benefits of exercise. My dad has always played tennis and skied, and he continues to in his 70s. When I was a kid he encouraged me to ski and play tennis as well. We also took Karate together. He didn't force me to exercise regularly, but he exposed me to the habit. In high school, I joined the track team and in college I joined a gym, and took dance lessons. I haven't skied, played tennis, or done Karate regularly in quite some time, but I did develop a habit of exercising regularly, and I have my dad to thank for that.

While doing research on the benefits of exercise, I found an article that discussed a study conducted in England that found that the cells of people who exercised appeared up to nine years younger than the cells of non-exercisers. Their findings suggested that exercising may protect the body against the aging process on a molecular level. So get moving if you haven't already begun an exercise program, and keep it up, if you have.

The one form of exercise that I've done consistently for over 20 years now is walking. I've done other things, too, but walking is the one thing I have *always* done.

I tried running and found it was a lot better for weight loss than walking, but for me, it led to injuries, mostly chronically sore knees.s Everyone I know who is a runner and has run over a period of several years has eventually complained of pains in their knees, hips, ankles or feet. Running is great in many ways, and I do recommend it, but in my experience it's hard on the body when done for a long time.

I did hear a story on NPR recently that said that running injuries are *not* inevitable. Some people can run their entire lives and never hurt themselves. Personally, though, I've not met a runner who has never complained of pains, at least occasionally. But I believed the story. There probably are life long runners whose bodies have thrived all along. I have to admit, I did know a man in his 90s who'd run the LA Marathon some 30-plus times, and he told me he ran every day. When I met him he was 93 and had great energy and vitality. So, for some, it really is great.

If you're a runner and it's working for you, that's awesome and of course you'll continue to enjoy it for as long as you can. But if you're considering what kind of regular exercise to do for the next 30, 40 years or more, I would recommend walking, because it seems to be less stressful on the joints. You might get sore if you're walking on concrete all the time, but if you wear proper shoes and you can find a track or hiking trail or beach, your knees and hips shouldn't suffer. You'll have to supplement walking with weight training and stretching in order to get and keep a fabulous body, but regular walking will help you stay young looking.

How much depends on you. I recommend at least 30 minutes 4 times a week, but more is even better. An hour a day would be great. Listen to your favorite music while you walk or do affirmations, meditate or pray. Try to walk fast enough to get your heart rate up higher than normal.

Regular exercise benefits the brain as well as the body. And since walking is easy and inexpensive, it is something one can always do. If you live in a climate that isn't conducive to walking, try finding an indoor track or a mall with long stretches of hallway.

According to an article called "The Effects of Exercise on the Brain," by MK McGovern, exercise leads to the release of neurotransmitters in the brain that alleviate pain, physical as well as mental. Also, exercise assists the brain in generating new neurons. *New neurons.* This suggests to me, that exercise is regenerative, meaning it creates something new in us. I equate "new" with youth. If walking regularly helps me make new neurons, my brain is therefore younger than if I sat on my butt and had nothing but "old neurons" to work with!

Weights

I workout with weights and on weight machines at the gym two to three times a week. On the weight training days, I usually skip the walking, because of time limitation. Supplementing your walking routine (or other aerobic exercise that gets your heart rate up) with weight training will keep you leaner than the walking (cardio) alone.

As you've probably heard before, weight training leads to more muscle mass and more muscle mass leads to a faster metabolism that helps you lose weight, because muscle burns more calories than fat. Careful, though, because you may think you can eat more because you've worked out, but if you eat too much more, more calories than you burn, it doesn't matter that you're exercising. You will still gain weight. I learned this the hard way. I went through a period wherein I was lifting weights quite a lot, but doing less walking (cardio) than usual. Indeed, I added muscle and looked pretty good, but I was eating more than usual, too, thinking I could, because muscle burns more calories than fat. I put on 10 pounds in just a few months! It looked much better than 10 pounds of fat would have looked, but I decided to watch my food intake more carefully and bring my weight back down. You will have to find what works best for your body. I recommend at least 30 minutes of cardio 4 times per week and 45 minutes to an hour of strength training 2 to 3 times per week. Develop the habit of working out consistently in your 20s and 30s and when you hit your 40s, 50s, and older, your body will look tighter, more defined, and years younger.

If you're already in your 40s or 50s, it's definitely not too late to begin a weight-training program. Start now and you will reap the benefits of aging better. Weight training increases bone mass, which helps ward off post-menopausal osteoporosis. Strength training also helps bones retain calcium, which also helps prevent osteoporosis.

Studies have shown that even elderly people can increase their bone density with weight training, so it really is never too late to start.

Increased bone density and improved muscle strength will assist you in keeping good posture and maintaining balance, which will help you move with the grace and confidence of a young person well into advanced years.

Water

As I've mentioned in other sections, drinking a lot of water has benefits that keep you young looking. It hydrates your skin, helping it look more plump and radiant. Drinking water also helps reduce hunger. Sometimes when we think we're hungry, we're really thirsty. Water also enhances fat loss. When you drink enough water, your kidneys and liver are aided in working to their full potential because the water assists them in flushing out the body's waste. When the kidneys don't receive enough water to work properly, the liver has to help, and then the liver is unable to perform its other functions properly, which causes fat loss to be delayed. Drinking water helps the body to function efficiently which leads to a higher metabolic rate, which leads to calories being burned faster. So drink up!

The combination of consistent walking, weight training and drinking plenty of water will help greatly in maintaining your weight. Weight maintenance is so helpful in aging well. Constantly fluctuating weight is stressful on the body. Maintaining a healthy weight is one of the best things you can do to stay young looking.

STAIR CLIMBING

Last year, I injured my shoulder while lifting weights. There was period of a few months, wherein, I couldn't use weight machines, because it was just too painful. It's amazing how involved the shoulder is a variety of activities.

During that time, I had a conversation with my friend Shelley and I told her I was worried about not being able to weight train. I feared my body would lose its definition. As it turned out, Shelley, who's about my age, had just been told by her doctor that *stair climbing* was the best exercise she could do. When I asked her why, she explained that it gives you a great calorie burn—about 5 to 7 calories a minute, depending on your weight. And it's very effective for improving bone density. Research shows that you can stimulate bone growth when you engage in activities, like stair climbing that put stress on the bones. This is particularly important for women close to menopause or in menopause, because bone density tends to decrease with declining estrogen levels.

I began reading up on stair climbing and found a number of articles quoting doctors who advised that climbing stairs regularly can increase aerobic capacity and bone density, reduce cholesterol, and improve muscle strength and stamina.

I began climbing up and down the six flights of stairs in the parking structure at my gym. I'd bring my ipod and listen to music while climbing for 15 minutes. That was all I could do at first. At the end of those 15 minutes, I'd been drenched with sweat! It's challenging and really gets your heart and lungs pumping. An unexpected benefit was that my skin began to look more vibrant due to an improvement in my circulation. I kept at it and now, months later, I can do 30 minutes. It's still challenging. I continue to sweat and get a bit breathless, but I'm inspired to keep it up, because I see benefits.

I stair climb two to three times per week for 25—30 minutes, alternating it with my walking days, and I've been doing this for a few months now. In that time, I've grown fitter, with a tighter butt and slimmer thighs. I've also noticed a reduction in belly fat. I'm convinced that stair climbing is a great fat-burner.

Another great thing about stair climbing is that it's free. You don't need a gym membership, you just need to find a flight of stairs. And you don't need any special equipment. It's a great addition to whatever fitness program you're already doing. And if you begin in your 40s or before and keep it up, it will help you avoid osteoporosis down the line. Keeping your bones healthy will contribute greatly to a youthful appearance as you get older.

STRETCH

As we grow older, our bodies become less flexible, but you can combat that stiffness if you stretch regularly. I have to admit I don't stretch as often as I should. I try to stretch after every weight training session, but I don't always succeed. Working on that, though, because I see the benefits that being limber has on a woman's beauty. There are two women I know, both older than I am, whose carriage I envy. Both of them have leaner limbs and stand a bit straighter than I do.

One is a lady who has practiced yoga for over 50 years. She has children who are in their 50s. Her body is astonishing—she's slim, her posture is excellent, and she carries herself with the swagger of a woman half her age.

The other is a cousin who's in her early 50s who has been taking ballet classes for 20 years. She does it for exercise and pleasure, not because she aspires to be a professional dancer. Though she began practicing late in life, for a ballet dancer, she nonetheless has the body of a 25 year old—an extraordinarily lean 25 year old. Her looks inspire admiration and appreciation in her husband. From what I've seen when in their presence, he is as proud of her body as she is!

Both ballet and yoga include lots of stretching and both result in a limber body. I am not good at either of them, unfortunately, but if you're attracted to practicing one or the other, I highly recommend both as an exercise you can do well into old age. Every woman I know who does yoga or ballet regularly has a spectacular body. Every one. But if you can't seem to get into either activity, like me, at least stretch regularly. Seriously. Stiffness is associated with old age. You absolutely *must* stretch and remain limber if you wish to age well. And isn't the idea of stretching a metaphor for lasting youth? We must always stretch ourselves to continue to live an invigorating life. If we rigidly stay the same and never stretch and grow, we become stiff and stagnant. So, stretch your body. Stretch your mind. Stretch in life, always reaching beyond where you've been.

MASSAGE

In my early 20s, I began seeing a chiropractor in New York. I had chronic back pain, probably from carrying too much stuff all during high school and college. Each visit included a 20-minute massage with a licensed massage therapist prior to the doctor's adjustment. I really didn't notice any benefit to my looks back then. But boy did I fall in love with massages. I continued to get them as the years went by.

In my mid 30s, I started getting shiatsu massages about once a month. Shiatsu is a Japanese form of massage that uses deep pressure along points in the body to balance one's energy. After the first few sessions I noticed that my skin seemed to look better the following day. When I mentioned this to the massage therapist, she explained that the shiatsu aided circulation. When blood circulation is increased it brings oxygen to the cells, which helps to improve the texture and tone of the skin.

Making massage a regular part of your beauty routine, year after year, will help your skin to age more gracefully.

According to an article in *Newsweek* Magazine, "Five Surprising Benefits of Massage" by Temma Ehrenfeld, massage may boost immunity because it helps reduce the level of cortisol in the body. Ehrenfeld also claims that studies suggest massage reduces hypertension as well. Stress and hypertension certainly contribute to aging, so if massage can reduce their effects, then it also helps to slow the process.

There isn't conclusive evidence to support the benefit of one type of massage over another, according to Ehrenfeld's article, so enjoy Swedish, deep tissue, or any kind you prefer. If the cost of a professional massage is prohibitive, you can still reap benefits by self-massaging parts of your own body: your hands, feet, arms and legs. Or try trading massages with a partner.

Make massage a habitual part of your health maintenance routine and you'll look and feel better.

SLEEP

Sufficient sleep is essential for looking young. I've had the luxury of working from home for most of the last 15 years and I have not had children, so, I've almost always been able to get as much sleep as I need. I realize this is not typical, and not everyone can sleep as late or as much as they'd like to. Still, everyone can try, to the best of their ability, to make a good night's sleep a habit and a priority. Certainly, if you're in your 20s and don't have kids yet, take advantage of the luxury of plenty of sleep while you're able to. Young women who hang out all night partying may be having a ball, but they won't look better for it.

Years ago my girlfriend Tracy had a difficult pregnancy wherein she had mandatory bed rest for the final few months. She told me that she looked about 10 years younger after getting all that rest. I never forgot that. There is a clear correlation between sleep and how we look. When we haven't slept in a couple of days, we look and feel awful. But what if we make it a long-term habit to get good sleep? In my experience, when a woman does cultivate that habit, she ages better than those who don't get adequate sleep.

The brain needs sleep to function properly. A sleep-deprived brain will result in disorientation equivalent to a person who is drunk. We know that the brain can affect all the other parts of the body, so if the brain isn't getting what it needs in terms of sleep, then the rest of the body is going to be adversely affected as well.

As women reach middle age and older, sleep disruption often occurs. Still, there are things you can do to improve the amount of time you're able to sleep. Be sure to use shades and curtains in your bedroom to keep morning sun from waking you too early. Try a sleep mask if you are sensitive to light. Earplugs are helpful if you're easily disturbed by noise. Reduce caffeine in your diet. And don't ingest anything with caffeine late in the day. If your mattress is no longer comfortable, replace it. Any adjustment you can make to help you sleep better and longer will benefit you.

A study cited in an article called, "How Sleep Affects Your Longevity," not only found a definite correlation between sleep and longevity, but it also suggested that by getting enough sleep each night we can control the advance of aging. The article says that if one does nothing else to ensure aging well, getting enough sleep should be the top priority.
During sleep the body rejuvenates itself; our cells are repaired.

According Dr. Perricone, anti-aging specialist and author of *The Wrinkle Cure*, it's essential to get enough sleep if you want to maintain a youthful appearance. Perricone explains that when we get good sleep, the body releases a youth hormone called "human growth hormone," that builds us up, rather than breaking us down, and it leads to increased muscle mass, thicker skin and stronger bones.

Good sleep habits, long term, will definitely help combat aging and assist you in staying healthier.

CAREFUL *HOW* YOU SLEEP

I have a terrible habit of sleeping on the right side of my face, which squishes my cheek into my pillow. In my 30s, I would wake up with a deep crease on that cheek, right along the nasolabial fold or laugh line. By the time I hit my 40s that crease became a permanent line. Of course I have combated it, to the best of my ability, with the skin brushing, moisturizing, etc. but it's still more pronounced than I'd like. For those of you reading this who still have time to avoid creating wrinkles that could have been prevented, please take heed and try to *learn to sleep on your back.*

I so wish I had cultivated the ability to lie on my back through the night when I was younger. That deep line is one of the only signs of my real age. Learning to sleep on your back will be a blessing for your face. In that position, everything on your face falls in the proper place so that the skin is smooth. If you can keep that position year after year, it will help to delay the aging process by not creating any new wrinkles.

SEX

A few years ago I traveled with my mother and a friend of hers to visit a friend of theirs who was in her 70s. Immediately, I noticed something different about this friend's energy. I'll call her Claire. Claire wasn't super slim, but she confidently wore a sleeveless top and it looked appealing on her. Her hair was a little longer than most women I knew in that age range and it skimmed her shoulders sensually. She wore a skirt that showed off her shapely calves, and skimpy sandals that boasted pretty, manicured toenails. She was, at 70-something, sex-y! No one had to tell me that this woman was still sexually active, and if anyone tried to tell me she wasn't, I wouldn't have believed them. I can't say for sure that she was having sex with a partner, but I strongly suspect she was. She was definitely in touch with her sexuality and it gave her the feminine, sparkly energy of a woman half her age. I studied her and made a note to myself that I'd be like that in my senior years.

According to an article by the editors of *Prevention,* one study showed that being sexually active on a regular basis can make you look up to 12 years younger.

Sex is healthy. Human connection, touching, emotional closeness—all of this is beneficial for our health and wellbeing. But even if you don't have a partner, you can still be sexually active, and you should be.

Masturbation is an awkward subject for many people, but if you don't have a lover, it can be a great way to stay in touch with your sexuality and improve your health. Bringing one's self to orgasm is a great stress reliever. The body releases endorphins during orgasm and they have a calming effect, which can help you sleep. As we know, good sleep helps you look younger.

Humans are sexual beings and if we don't have the opportunity for a sexual outlet, then we're suppressing a part of ourselves, and that causes blocked energy. Blocked energy stagnates us. Energy is supposed to flow.

With or without a partner, be good to yourself sexually. Enjoy your body, appreciate it, and treat yourself to the release of orgasms regularly. If you don't have a partner, fantasize and visualize the best kind of sexual experience you can possibly imagine. Smile. Enjoy it. Feel the love, the heat, the passion. Enjoy and honor your body. It's good for you, your energy, and your looks.

If you do have a sex partner and the sex is not great, relax, have fun, focus on gratitude and appreciation. Don't take it so seriously, just connect and express and receive love.

If the connection is not healthy or loving, let it go. Get out. Move on. Don't let fear keep you in an unhealthy relationship of any kind. The only thing to fear is remaining unhappy, because if you do that, your energy won't allow you to attract all the good you deserve. Don't fear letting go. If you let go, something is going to fill that space. And you can create a better experience. Being alone for a time can be better than being in bad company. And if you believe there's someone else for you, that person will show up. I speak from experience.

If your sex life with a partner is good, well, hallelujah! There are wonderful benefits in addition to those I've already mentioned. The physical act can get your heart rate up, reduce your appetite, burn calories, stretch your limbs, boost self-esteem and strengthen the immune system. According to an article on *WEB* MD, "10 Surprising Health Benefits of Sex," by Kathleen Doheney, having sex regularly has been linked with higher levels of the antibody immunoglobulin A, which can protect you from getting colds and infections. Just the touching alone is healing and comforting, and can leave you feeling more relaxed and confident, which shows up nicely on your face, body and in your essence as a more beautiful, radiant energy. If you're *in love* with your partner, then the benefits are further enhanced. When the physical connection is compounded with a deeply emotional one, you're moved and gratified on levels that we probably can't even measure, but you know the difference when you feel it. If someone has ever told you that you're "glowing," you were probably having good sex with someone you were in love with.

The great news is we can keep that glow even as we age. I've seen it for myself in people in their 70s and even 80s! So, make sexual health and happiness a priority, because it's fun, good for you, and definitely helps keep your energy vibrant and young.

CLEARING OLD EMOTIONS – CRY IT OUT

A few years ago, I took a spiritual writing class with my friend Dena Crowder, a wonderful teacher, healer and practical mystic based in the Los Angeles area. She told us a story about a marvelously beautiful and youthful woman she'd met who was in her 50s. In the story, a man was introduced to the woman and subsequently awed by her. He was aware of her real age, but remarked with astonishment that she looked, "so much younger," and that she was "radiant." He wanted to know why. Why did she look so much younger than other women her age?

The woman responded that she had cried for two years. He looked confused. She went on to explain that several years earlier, she had gone through a period where she spent many months crying every day, grieving and releasing all kinds of old emotional wounds and resentments, and she did it until it was done. It took two years. She functioned, albeit minimally. As I understood it, she worked, paid her bills, but spent most of her free time alone, dealing with the emotional work she had decided she must do.

The result turned out to be rejuvenating. Inner peace came with the release of that emotional darkness and it was like clouds dissipating, letting the sunshine through. She was radiant, because there was nothing blocking her inner light. She had worked through everything that had wounded her in her life.

Most of us certainly don't have the luxury of taking two years to cry. But we can apply the idea of releasing old wounds and resentments, and do it in a way that works within our lives.

Much of what we get angry, frustrated or sad about in our present circumstance has a relationship to past events that have resulted in our feeling angry, frustrated or sad. So, when we respond with an emotion to something in the present, we are, in a sense, recalling previous events where our emotional reaction was the same. Often the event in our present, that we *think* we're so upset about, is merely a trigger causing us to re-experience the past. If we can go back and work through the original event, release it, forgive it, and make peace with it, we'll be free not to have to respond with such intensity in the present.

Sure, people may still annoy you or hurt your feelings in the moment, but if you work out the deeper source of your pain, you will no longer react as intensely, for as long, or as often as you do when old wounds are left festering.

That's what this woman did. She revisited events that had left her with emotional scars and she consciously released them. Many of us make the mistake of allowing pain to stick with us. We don't have to do that. Of course, some things are incredibly painful and take time to recover from, but we *can* recover. Some people choose not to. They would prefer to live as if the pain was an integral part of their spirit. It is not. The spirit is resilient. We can move through pain.

We can look at things that cause us pain and with time, choose to stop giving energy to them. If pain persists, allow the grief to come up, but then choose to let it go. I know that this is far easier said than done, but it can be done.

Forgive

Release every circumstance and every person that has caused you pain. Make a list of everything and everyone that you can think of and then go down that list and forgive and let go. Even if they really don't deserve it. Even if they are jerks. It doesn't matter. It isn't about them, it's about *you*. You don't forgive them because they were right to harm you. You don't forgive them in order to be in denial about what they did. And you don't do it to say that the hurt you've suffered was okay. You forgive to heal yourself, to move on and to free up your energy. You do it to make your life happier.

This is not generally something one can do quickly or easily. But I've found that once I commit to this type of emotional release work, experiencing forgiveness happens more freely.

It took me many years to forgive someone that I felt had wronged me. I was committed to that person being wrong, committed to being angry and no one could tell me that I should stop feeling the way I did. But eventually, I figured out that the resentment I was holding was causing *me*, not the other person, harm. Nothing good was coming of it. It was negatively affecting choices I was making. It was keeping a cloud over my life. When it became apparent that it was a hindrance, I decided I wanted to let it go. But I couldn't. I didn't know how.

Forgiveness is a process, and it can take longer than we'd like. But it began when I made the choice to do it. I tried everything. I prayed, went to church, went to therapy, read self-help books, did hypnosis, affirmations—whatever I could think of. Little by little, over time, I worked on releasing it. Ultimately, what I did was transcend it. I looked at what I'd perceived had been done to me from a broader, spiritual perspective. After several years had passed, I was able to see how I'd developed as a result of what had hurt me. I'd become stronger, more evolved, more compassionate and wiser. From that vantage point, I saw how what had seemed to break me, had *not* broken me. I was finally able to appreciate it as a part of my life's journey, and as an experience that, ultimately, made me a better person. After a while it dissipated and was gone. What replaced it was energy-- a more vibrant energy of love and happiness.

You must *want* to let go of resentment in order to release it. You must decide you are going to do it. It is a choice. The emotional release won't always happen right away, but if you commit to your wellbeing, and you consciously heal old emotional wounds, you will cleanse your spirit and eventually transform that negativity into peace. Wanting to let it go is the first step. Surrender and ask God, the Universe, your higher self, or whatever makes sense to you, to assist you and you will succeed in that transformation. And the result will be a brighter, more beautiful, and more youthful you.

CLEAR OLD JUNK FROM YOUR LIVING SPACE

It may not seem logical that removing old stuff from your surroundings would have any effect on your appearance. But everything is made up of energy, including people, and our energy is affected by our surroundings. I'm not saying that if you clean the trash and dust from under your bed you're going to have fewer wrinkles the next day. What I am saying is that if you clean the trash and dust from under your bed, you will have created a space for better energy flow and that will eventually positively affect your own energy. When your energy is better, you feel better and your looks reflect that.

It might be unconscious, but when you put a little effort into renewing your environment by getting rid of old, useless possessions that are no longer serving you, the energy is transformed in a beneficial way. You create a space wherein your vibration can be at its finest.

Old junk has stagnant energy. Our goal, if our aim is to be youthful, should be to surround ourselves with things that reflect our aliveness and vitality. Of course it's okay to keep old things that are beautiful or dear to us, or that we are getting use out of. It's not, however, a good idea to keep anything that isn't beautiful, special, meaningful, needed, or useful in some way.

Clear unwanted, unneeded things out of your living space and you will make room for the energy of new things that bring you joy. On a subconscious level, this type of renewal will energize you. Over time, if you regularly purge your space of all that is old and not useful, this will assist you in creating the energy of youthful vitality.

ADD SOME LIFE TO YOUR LIVING SPACE

I believe that having live things in our environment has a positive effect on us. My preference is green plants; I find them soothing, nurturing and energizing. Plants also benefit us by helping to filter the air.

Breathing cleaner, purer air helps us feel better, which makes us more vibrant. And looking at plants, even artificial plants, positively affects us psychologically. Their vibration has the energy of life! Plants inspire me. I would much rather spend my days in a plant-filled room than one without any. I draw energy from them, and I believe I am more vibrant, when in their presence.

What you draw energy from day in and out will be specific to you. But to assist you in maintaining a youthful, vibrant energy, I recommend surrounding yourself with things that make you feel alive. Consider the energy of fountains, candles, wind chimes, art, photographs, quality furniture, fixtures and the colors on your walls. Anyplace where you spend a lot of time will have an effect on your energy, which can positively or negatively affect your appearance.

If you spend time in a place for a number of years, the effects increase exponentially. The energy of the space becomes a part of you. So, be purposeful about what surrounds you. Let it inspire healthy, youthful, vibrant, energetic feelings in you and you will reap the benefits.

GET OUT IN NATURE WHEN YOU CAN

Perhaps you live in a city without much access to nature. Or maybe nature doesn't interest you all that much. If not, have you ever considered the benefits of trees and green space to a person's wellbeing? They are numerous and include purified air and a greater sense of peace.

If you live within access to green space, good for you! Enjoy it! Take a drive or walk, or a hike. Spend time around trees. Or if you live near a body of water, enjoy that, too. Both green space and lakes, rivers and oceans, have energy that feeds us in a positive way. For some people, the beach is the best balm to a stressed-out psyche. For others, it's being in the mountains, the woods, or a park or field. Whatever it is for you, be sure to give yourself some time to connect with the beauty of nature. It will have a positive effect on your energy and thus on your appearance. If you make it a habit to recharge in nature regularly, it will penetrate your psyche in an energizing way and assist you in vibrating youth.

If you don't live near green space, perhaps you can you create it. Plant some trees or flowers near your home or apartment. Or get a potted tree or even a few of them and create a green oasis on your patio or in your living room. Plant a garden or start or join a community garden.

There's something very energizing about growing things. I love to garden. Digging in the earth, planting things and watching them grow helps keep me young because it creates good, vibrant energy— the energy of life.

I recommend that you make it a habit to spend time in nature weekly, or at the least, monthly. Whether it's the beach, mountains, a park, or your own yard, be there long enough to take in the sights, sounds, smells and the vibration. It will become a part of you, and you'll carry that vibration of loveliness within you.

NON-TOXIC CLEANING

As I've said repeatedly, I believe that chemicals and toxins that get into our systems are harmful to us and contribute to aging. I would encourage you to consider ways in which you can minimize the toxins you come into contact with through eating, breathing or touching.

Cleaning products are usually filled with chemical additives. When we spray industrial cleaner on our counter tops, in our bathrooms, on mirrors and walls, we inhale them. If we clean without rubber gloves, and they get onto our skin they can end up in our bloodstream.

Did you know that you can use white vinegar in place of window cleaner? It can also be used in place of antibacterial cleanser. You can add it to laundry, wipe counter tops down, or even use it to mop the floor. And the best part is, it's non-toxic. Don't worry about the sour smell of the vinegar. It dissipates quickly on hard surfaces and will not leave your home smelling like a salad.

Baking soda, also non-toxic, can be used to scour sinks and tubs. You may also use it to clean stovetops or scrub toilets. And baking soda, like vinegar, can be added to laundry to get it brighter.

If you mix baking soda AND vinegar, you'll have a super cleaning duo. Sprinkle baking soda on a counter top or in the sink. Put white vinegar into a spray dispenser and spray on the baking soda. It reacts with bubbles and will deep clean just about everything.

If you use baking soda and white vinegar in place of store bought cleaners, you will not inhale harmful fumes while cleaning. And if the baking soda and vinegar come in contact with your skin, it will not introduce harmful chemicals into your body.

Cleaning this way is better for you and for your environment. It will reduce your exposure to the toxic chemicals found in everyday cleaning products, which, over time, can have an adverse effect on health and, in turn, contribute to aging. Don't believe *me*? Anti-aging experts Dr. Oz and Michael Roizen wrote a book called *You: Staying Young: The Owner's Manual for Extending Your Warranty* and there is a chapter devoted to non-toxic cleaning. They, too, caution their readers about the connection between toxins and aging.

I heard an interesting story on National Public Radio that covered a hotel chain's use of a revolutionary cleaning machine that used salt water as a cleanser. The people interviewed for the story included employees and their employer. The employer revealed that after introducing this cleanser that uses no cleaning chemicals other than salt water, the hotels maid staff had far fewer workers being injured and far fewer calling in with colds and other illnesses. The employees said they felt much better using the cleaner with the salt water than when they were using harsh chemicals everyday. This tells me that there is, indeed, a connection between store bought, industrial strength cleaners and health.

Since I don't know how to make the salt water cleaner, nor do I have access to the machine used to apply it, I can't pass this onto you. However, the point I'm trying to make is that there is empirical evidence that using cleaning products we could not safely ingest causes harm to our health. Conversely, using cleaning products that we *can* safely ingest, like salt, baking soda or vinegar, proves beneficial to health by reducing exposure to toxic chemicals.

Limiting exposure to toxic chemicals should be part of any anti-aging plan.

NOT TOXIC GARDENING

In the previous chapter I discussed how vinegar could be used for cleaning. Did you know that vinegar may also be used as a weed killer? Try it. You can pour it on weeds, avoiding grass, and the weed will shrivel and die within a day or two. Use enough vinegar to penetrate the soil, so the root receives it as well. You can also spray vinegar on the spaces in your driveway where grass and weeds crop up.

Vinegar is so much better for the environment than poisonous weed killer. Anything you put into or onto your soil will eventually work its way into ground springs that eventually connect to larger sources of water because your lawn is a watershed.

A "watershed" is an area of land that drains down slope to the lowest point. Water moves through drainage pathways underground. These pathways converge into streams and rivers, eventually reaching the ocean. In cities like Los Angeles, where I live, storm drains lead water directly to the Pacific Ocean. This is why it's so important not to pollute our lawns and streets with trash and toxins, because they end up in the storm drains and flow to the ocean.

Ocean water evaporates, collecting in the atmosphere as clouds and eventually becomes rain. If we don't want toxic rain flowing down on us, we must do our part not to be polluters.

So, please don't add toxic chemicals to your lawn. Pull out weeds by hand or use vinegar to kill them.

Instead of chemical fertilizer, consider composting to make good soil to fertilize your lawns and gardens. This benefits the environment by recycling plant products and other things like egg shells and coffee grinds, creating less waste and also enriching the soil.

Worm composting, a little different from regular composting, will result in creating "worm tea," an amazing and effective fertilizer that when mixed with water will fertilize grass, plants and flowers. Worm tea also helps control yard insects. Using worm tea as a fertilizer and insecticide is a far healthier choice than store bought chemicals.

I'm going to refrain from giving a how-to on composting and worm composting, but if you're interested in natural, non-toxic gardening, please look further into it for yourself. There are plenty of articles online to help get you started with composting.

Creating healthy alternatives to benefit your lawn and garden will benefit your own health and your family's as well. Again, as we limit our exposure to toxins it benefits our long-term health and help us to age better.

EXTRAS FOR THOSE OVER 45

If you're reading this and you're in your 20s or 30s, you probably don't need the things I'm about to suggest. And if you don't need them, please don't use them, at least not until you reach a point where you really do.

Using the things I'm going to suggest directly contradicts what I said earlier about chemicals. I'm going to suggest some chemicals. And using them too soon in life will not benefit you. I've encouraged you to avoid chemicals and toxins, and I would like you to avoid them for as long as possible, because, in general, unnatural chemicals are not healthful and their use does not engender youth.

But once you reach your mid 40s a few things begin to happen that require the use of a couple of chemicals that can help you *look* younger, which will help you *feel* younger. When you feel younger, you carry yourself in a more youthful way and that can help you look younger, too.

Age spots and discoloration due to sun sensitivity begins to be more pronounced in one's 40s. For me, it happened ever earlier, in my late 30s. The very slightest sun exposure would result in hyper-pigmentation on my face. Even though I was already wearing hats to protect my skin, if a bit of sun managed to hit me, which occurred mostly when I was wearing ball caps, I actually started to look "dirty" from sunspots. Once a friend told me it looked like there was a smudge of newspaper ink above my lip. It turned out to be discoloration from UV rays. Not very attractive!

Hydroquinone

An esthetician recommended a product containing hydroquinone that fades dark spots. I was familiar with hydroquinone, because as an acne sufferer, I had marks left by pimples. My dermatologist had prescribed the hydroquinone product, Eldoquin Forte, but I'd only used it temporarily. Once my acne was under control, I did not wish to continue using it. A few years later, however, when my skin had become more mature, dark spots and blotches began appearing even where there had been no blemishes! And so it was time to revisit the idea, and the use of hydroquinone.

I do not believe hydroquinone is "healthy." I do not recommend it if you don't really need it to even out your skin tone. If you can use other remedies with similar results, such as Vitamin C, by all means, use them. But nothing works for me as well as products with hydroquinone.

The brand I like most is a gel called DermaClair. Like most over the counter remedies, it contains 2% hydroquinone. (Products containing 4%, like Eldoquin Forte, require a prescription.) This product, which I use at night under coconut oil, fades discolorations and gives me wonderfully even-toned skin.

I can't, in good conscience *highly* recommend it, because I can't tell you that it is good for you, and because I really don't believe in putting things on your skin that you could not safely ingest. You certainly would not eat hydroquinone. But I would like you to have the information and be able to try it, if you chose, because it has worked for me.

Animal studies where high doses have been administered have shown the potential of hydroquinone to cause cancer. I believe the doses used in the studies were far greater than one would use on their skin, but nonetheless, you should be aware of the risks.

Yet, I must be honest with you, my skin looks younger and has a glow as a result of using this product.

While I am conflicted about this contradiction in my "toxin-free" philosophy, I've realized, as I've gotten older, that things are usually not entirely one way or the other. An approach to health and beauty can be as complex as life itself. I've made peace with the contradiction and believe it's okay to be 95% chemical free, and use a few things that may not be free of toxins, if they work well.

Periodically, I check for studies on hydroquinone and according to what I've read, the product has been used for decades. Although when used in very high concentrations it was shown to cause cancer in mice, that is, apparently, *not* confirmation that moderate use will cause cancer in humans. I've not seen any articles or studies that have found hydroquinone to cause cancer in humans.

The choice is yours. If you have not yet experienced the aging look of blotchy, hyper-pigmented skin, then you should avoid hydroquinone. But if you have noticed new dark spots and patches of discoloration popping up on your once even-toned skin, you may be feeling unhappy about the way you look and you may feel that you have no control over it. If this is the case, begin wearing hats and sunscreen, if you don't already do so, and try applying hydroquinone to the spots at night before bed. It will take a few weeks before the dark areas begin to fade, but they will. Once faded, you can stop using the product, but you must keep your face protected from the sun, or the spots will return.

Minoxidil

As a woman enters her mid-40s and goes through peri-menopause, she may notice that her hair has begun to thin. This can be deeply traumatic. I know it was for me. While I wasn't always a huge fan of my naturally curly, unruly hair, I did appreciate that it covered my entire head! My hair had always been thick, something I lamented when I tried to straighten it with blow-dryers and hot irons.

One day, I blew my hair straight and noticed that it looked very thin at the crown, along the back of my part. I had a round bald spot there! This resulted in a full-blown anxiety attack. I was on my way to an important meeting and no matter which way I brushed my hair or shifted my part, I could not cover that spot. It was awful. I felt completely unattractive and insecure. I can barely remember the meeting, and nothing came of it, because I was preoccupied with my hair-loss problem.

Shortly afterwards, I went to my doctor to discuss it. I tend to have recurring anemia. He told me that the lack of iron in my blood could contribute to hair loss. Because I prefer a mostly plant-based diet, it doesn't appeal to me to eat red meat, but I *did* begin eating it. Being bald felt worse than eating animals. My anemia did improve, but my hair loss continued.

I did not like the idea of trying Minoxidil. Despite my use of hydroquinone, I continued, and still continue, to resist the idea of putting unnecessary chemicals on my skin. But I was going *bald!* If it could help me, it *was* necessary.

I began using generic Minoxidil for women. I used it for about three or four months before I really noticed a change. It wasn't significant, but it was something, so I was encouraged. At least my hair seemed to be falling out less.

Then one day I had coffee with my beautiful friend, Lucia. When I relayed my ordeal to her, she told me that she had a few women friends who were experiencing the same issue. Some of these women were young—in their 20s. She'd learned from a dermatologist that despite the caveats that women should avoid the men's formula, women actually *can* use the "extra strength for men" formula with no adverse effects. And another tip from her dermatologist: the "generic" version is every bit as effective as the name brand, yet far less expensive.

Since I was having only moderate success with the women's formula, I decided to try it. It changed my life. I have been using the 5% "extra strength for men" formula for several months now and that unsightly bald spot has completely filled in. I am so grateful. The value of confidence cannot be overstated and having my hair back has restored that confidence.

Here's an extra bit of information that you might not know: If your eyebrows are thin in spots or uneven, Minoxidil can be applied to grow them in more fully as well.

Eyebrows that are too thin can make you look older. Full brows are a hallmark of youth, so if you've plucked yours super thin you may want to consider growing them in a bit fuller. You can put a few drops of the Minoxidil on a cotton swab and rub it over the areas around your brow that you'd like to fill in. It will take a couple of months, but eventually you'll see results.

Hair dye

Permanent hair color contains chemicals and so, it too, conflicts with my health principals. Studies have shown that long-term use of permanent hair dye can lead to bladder cancer. Dyes that wash out don't seem to show the same carcinogenic effects, so if you can use those, I'd recommend them over permanent dye. Another benefit is that, because they wash out, you can apply them yourself if you want to, and save on costly salon visits.

Dyeing one's hair is not for everyone, and is even considered controversial, because it suggests women should feel the need to be inauthentic. But how can one share information about looking youthful without mentioning the difference covering one's gray can make in appearance?

Some women like the look of their gray hair. And on some, it's beautiful. If you're one of those, congratulations. Enjoy your gray. For most women, though, gray hair really does make them look older. I saw a photograph of my stunningly beautiful sister when she'd reached her early 50s, and she was gray at her temples. I couldn't believe the picture, because she did not look like my sister. The photo, with all that gray, made her look like a much older lady.

Recently, I spent some time with my sister. She has covered her gray with a beautiful, rich brown. She's in her mid 50s and without the gray she looks like she's in her 30s. We were on vacation and went to an African-American museum together in Jacksonville, Florida, and she requested a senior discount. The ticket saleswoman was taken aback. She demanded to see I.D. and when my sister produced it, she was shocked. She called her co-worker over so that together they could marvel at how this youthful, stunning woman was actually a senior. Hair color can make a huge difference that goes even beyond the look of your hair. If you look in the mirror and appear younger, you feel better, and you'll exude more youth and confidence, which enhances your overall vibration.

So, don't feel you have to age gracefully and allow the gray to come in, unless that's really what you want. If what you really want is to look and feel young, don't be too proud to cover up what doesn't support that image.

MEDITATION

Maintaining youth may not be the first thing that comes to mind when we think about meditating. Generally, the desired benefits of meditation are based in spirituality—inner peace—not vanity. Meditation helps to create a more vibrant mind and soul. I believe that a byproduct of those is a more vibrant energy and appearance as well.

One of the things that contributes to aging is stress. When you get stressed and have no skills to combat it, over time, it's going to adversely affect your health, and ultimately your looks as well. You may develop frown or worry lines. Your anxiety may cause you to overeat or to eat the wrong things, or it may cause you to drink too much or to smoke. You may lose sleep, bite your nails, pull out your hair. Whatever way that stress manifests in your experience, it probably is not engendering youth and beauty.

Meditating regularly can help. There are many different approaches to meditation. You may have to try a variety of things before you find what works for you. My approach is different depending on my circumstances. Sometimes, I prepare for meditation. I turn the ringer off on the phone, light candles and sit on a pillow cross-legged on the floor. But sometimes, I need to meditate wherever I am: while waiting to go into a meeting, or waiting in the doctor's office, or even while stuck in traffic on the freeway.

Meditation is, essentially, quieting the mind enough to be still and peaceful. When you meditate you can try to think of nothing at all, or you might think of a mantra, or affirmation that appeals to you. If you wish meditation to enhance your looks and health, you might choose an affirmation such as: "I am happy, healthy and beautiful. All is well in my world." Or you can affirm something more specific, like: "My skin is clear and radiant."

Even if you meditate in ways that have no direct connection to your health and beauty, your health and beauty will be enhanced. Quieting the mind, taking time for yourself, bringing peace into your experience cannot help but benefit your health. And the serenity you create will show up on you in a lovely way as well. Look at the expression of someone who is stressed and overwhelmed and compare it to someone at peace. The repeated expression of stress on a face and body will, over time, age it. The repeated expression of peace on a face and body will, over time, create loveliness.

VISUALIZATION

A powerful way to assist in the accomplishment of our goals is to visualize them already achieved. If you decide to commit to a lifestyle that helps to maintain a healthy, youthful appearance, you might picture yourself slim, glowing, active, attractive, happy, energetic etc., the way you imagine you'll be once you have done all the work it takes to get there. By combining visualization with all the other things recommended in this book, you will see results faster. And as you visualize, try to feel happy and excited about the results you're seeing. The better it feels as you visualize and the more passionate you are, the more quickly you will manifest results.

Close your eyes and relax. Get comfortable either sitting or reclining. See yourself looking, feeling, as you wish to be.

You may have an event you're preparing for, such as a reunion or a wedding. See yourself at the event looking spectacular: gorgeous, slim, far younger than your age. Picture your face smooth and clear, your hair shiny and full, and your body in amazing shape. See yourself at the event being happy, enjoying a great time. Imagine the very best possible scenario.

Another way you can use visualization is to collect photographs or cut them from magazines when you see something that you like and would like to have or emulate. You can create a vision board with these images. For example, if you see someone with the kind of body you'd like to have, you might cut out the photo and replace the head with a photo of your own. Or if you see a hairstyle or kind of hair you'd like, you might cut it out and paste it on your vision board.

As you add to the board, be sure that the images don't contradict one another. You might like a short hairstyle and a long one, but if you put both images on the board, you're unlikely to create or attract either, because they conflict. Be clear about what you want.

Put the vision board somewhere that you'll see it often. Or take a few minutes each day to look at the board and then close your eyes and imagine yourself with the things you've chosen. This is a powerful tool to help you achieve your health and beauty goals.

OPTIMISM

One of the best things you can do to improve the quality of your health and looks is to *believe* that you can, in fact, improve the quality of your health and looks. If you don't think that anything you try will work, you're probably right. Attitude contributes greatly to the probability of success.

I believe that in order to change, we must allow ourselves shifts in consciousness. If you're in your 20s or 30s, try to cultivate a propensity to expect the best. I wish someone had persuaded me to do so when I was young. I tended to feel undeserving of good things and I also worried about all that might go wrong. If I'd known then what I know now, I would have turned my attention away from negative thinking, and I would have pictured all that could go *right*. That is what I recommend.

Our focus here is on health, beauty, and remaining youthful, and we can certainly assist ourselves in pursuing all three with an attitude of optimism. No matter what your circumstances at this moment, believe that it's possible for you to be healthier, more beautiful, and to feel and look younger. The mere act of opening your mind to these possibilities will help you create them in your experience.

If you find yourself expecting negative things, take a moment to stop and redirect your thoughts. Instead of worrying about all that might go wrong, think about all the good that could happen. This can be difficult if your tendency has been to think in negative ways, but you can change that. You can begin to talk to yourself when negative things come into your mind, and you can give your mind something better to focus on. Practice this each time you find sabotaging thoughts coming up. Give yourself a new, better thought, and you will get better and better at it, until it becomes a habit. One friend told me she had a phrase, "Cancel, cancel!" which she repeated to herself every time her thinking began to go awry. Find something you can say to yourself when you think a negative thought and practice expecting the best.

GRATITUDE

I vaguely remember seeing an episode of Oprah where she spoke of keeping a gratitude journal. And I watched the popular documentary, *The Secret* a number of times and noticed that gratitude came up a few times. It is said that one of the best ways to change your life for the better is to have gratitude. As you focus on it, more things to be grateful for occur in your life. This has been the case for me. I firmly believe that being in touch with gratitude constantly, or at least often, changes your energy. It improves it.

You are what you think about, so if you're thinking about all that you're dissatisfied with, that's what your energy is going to reflect. If you're thinking about things you appreciate, your energy is going to reflect beauty, because gratitude carries with it a lovely energy. Appreciation makes you smile inside and out. This benefits you in ways you can't see. Your body benefits when you're emitting an energy of gratitude. You're calmer, hopeful, happy, peaceful. This has a positive effect on the way you think and ultimately on the way you look.

Look at yourself in the mirror when you are angry, frustrated and miserable. Look at yourself in the mirror when you are peaceful and appreciative. What do you see? If you're a gorgeous person, okay, maybe you're still gorgeous whether you're happy or angry. But tension, which is inevitable when you're frustrated or angry, over time will be visible on your face and in your body and, over the years, it will age you and make you less attractive than if you cultivate the habit of being in gratitude and feeling peaceful and loving. Over the years, being grateful for things will give you a youthful loveliness that people who remain grumpy and frustrated simply cannot exude.

FOCUS ON YOURSELF, NOT ON CHANGING OTHERS

I have to admit, I've been guilty of spending copious amounts of energy contemplating what's wrong with others, and on trying to change them. If you've ever had a relationship with a partner, friend, parent or child, you've probably been guilty at some point too. I think it's nearly impossible to avoid *ever* trying to control a partner or trying to get them to behave in certain way, or to do what you want. A little bit of that is necessary at times, of course. What I'm talking about, though, is obsessing on another person's flaws to the degree that too much of your mental energy is wrapped up in that. If all or most of your energy is focused on someone else, and how they need to change, then you can't access that energy to further your own goals and purpose. As your energy is drained away from you, your youth and vitality are sucked away too!

If the relationship itself is more satisfying than accomplishing your own goals, then so be it. But if you're resenting something and you're frustrated, don't blame the other person and focus on how they're keeping you from accomplishing what you want to do. Find a way to move forward. Take your attention off what's wrong with them and do something constructive. Focusing on a friend or partner's problems to the point where you're immobile is a terrible way to spend your energy and your life. When you stop spending your energy trying to change others you'll have much more energy for your *own* use.

Say a friend or partner has a trait or a problem that affects you and the relationship in a negative way. Of course you want them to change the trait or the behavior. But you must determine if that is even within your power. Usually it is not. If the person does not want to change there is very little you can do to help them, or persuade them do so.

I'm not referring to minor things, like getting your husband to fix stuff around the house or getting your kid to stop doing things that annoy you, or getting your boyfriend to be more romantic, though these things can be energy drainers as well.

I'm talking about fundamental issues, things like substance abuse, infidelity, emotional unavailability, chronic inability to be responsible, chronic debting or under-earning, etc. If you think there is anything you can do to change a person who has these types of issues, you're probably wasting your time, energy and yes, your youth.

I'm not suggesting that you must leave the person (though that's not a bad idea if the behavior consistently makes your life unhappy), but if you're going to stay in the situation, you are better off accepting that this is who the person is. Find peace with that, rather than trying to change the person or hoping that they'll change. If you keep trying to change him (or her) and keep hoping that he'll change, you'll find yourself repeatedly disappointed.

When you find yourself emotionally engaged in this type of situation, try to disengage from complaining about them, or trying to control them, and focus your energy back on yourself. Ask yourself if this situation is similar to one you may have experienced in the past with someone else. If so, acknowledge that there is a pattern. There is a reason you have attracted this situation to yourself. Try to figure out what that reason is. What is it you would have to believe about yourself to draw a particular situation into your life time and time again? When you can identify what that is, you will then have some power over changing that belief about yourself.

For example, if you find yourself consistently drawn to men who criticize you, know that this is no coincidence. You are attracted, perhaps unconsciously, to critical people. Why? What would you have to believe about yourself that would draw one critical partner after another to you? Probably that you are not good enough and that you don't deserve to be treated with support and respect. So your task would be to re-train yourself to believe that you *are* good enough, and that you *are* worthy of loving, supportive behavior.

Rather than trying to force the person to stop criticizing you, as you change the belief about yourself and build your self esteem, you may find your own behavior changes, and that change in behavior leads to the transformation of the situation. When you build your self-esteem, you won't find the criticism as resonant as you previously had. You won't need it to confirm your negative feelings about yourself. This can't help but create a shift in the dynamic. As you change, the other person will have to adjust, but the only effective change you can make is within yourself.

This is just one example of how we engage in unproductive expenditures of energy within relationships, but there are many ways we do this. Only you can know the specific ways you participate in it. What I'd like to encourage you to do is to look at your own relationships and identify places where you are wasting your energy, because if you begin to draw that energy back to yourself, soon it will energize *you* and serve your goals and desires, which will spark your vitality and assist you in radiating a frequency of youth.

LEARN SOMETHING NEW

When we're young, we are constantly learning new things. Our brains are always challenged, developing, and bringing in more information. If you watch children at play, they enjoy discovering new things. I think it's our natural state, to be delighted by the stimulation of learning something we once did not know. It keeps our brains young and excited. There is always more to learn. We don't have to stop developing our minds or physical skills just because we reach middle age, or old age.

If you want to assist yourself in cultivating youth, learning new things is an essential part of that. Those new things can be intellectual or physical, preferably both. Our minds *and* our bodies benefit by being challenged.

Whatever it is you enjoy learning about, make a commitment to do some reading on the subject each week. Or if you've always wanted to develop the ability to swim, dance, sail, cook, sing, paint—whatever, sign up for a class. Or order some instructional videos or compact discs. Do what you can to nurture your innate desire to learn new things.

I recently decided to take Salsa lessons. For most of my life, I've believed that I could not learn to dance. I was simply not coordinated enough, and had no rhythm. Ironically, I've made a living by writing film and television projects about dance.

For much of my life, I've attended dance classes here and there, but I never felt good about dancing, because of a long held belief that I was predisposed to be terrible at it. I was a black girl who grew up in an all-white environment, and when I got around my relatives they teased me about dancing like a white girl. These days, that has no significance; White girls dance as well as anyone. But back in the 70s, it meant having no rhythm. I internalized the criticism and allowed it to define my ability.

One of the great things about getting older is that you learn that some of the things you once believed are not necessarily true. It was indeed true that I never became a good dancer. However, it is not true that I'm incapable of learning. So now, at 46, I'm learning and enjoying it. And I'm not only learning dance moves, but I'm learning about music as well. I'm learning how to find the beat. I'm being exposed to a new culture. All of this is mentally and physically stimulating. Bringing something new into my life fills me with excitement, and makes me feel young.

In our busy lives it's often difficult to introduce new things. Many of us are overwhelmed, over-scheduled, taking care of others, working etc. But if you plan ahead you *can* carve out an hour or two a week to devote to new learning. Look at your schedule and all the hours you have in the week, and pre-plan that time for yourself. On your drive to work, you might listen to language CDs in the car, or a novel, or non-fiction book. You might plan your family's weekend activity to include your new learning—go to a museum exhibit, or a play, a concert, or whatever interests you. Before bed during the week, you might watch a DVD on your subject of interest, or read up on your passion, or even practice it. You get the idea. Whatever it is that you're interested in, find some time to devote to cultivating your knowledge of it, even if it's just an hour a week.

Your body, mind and spirit will delight in the fact that you are nurturing yourself, and this will make your vibration sparkle and hum with vivaciousness and youth.

BE GOOD TO OTHERS

What do you think makes you happy? Is it looking good? Money? A relationship? I've spent many years contemplating how to be happy and what I've come to believe is that in order to be happy one must like herself (or himself). So how does a person develop self-love? I used to think it was about doing my best, accomplishing things and being successful. That helps. But when I'm truly happiest is when I am treating everyone the best way that I can. For me, one of the ways I do that is by enhancing my community. I've been an advocate for tree-planting where I live, because I believe that trees benefit people's physical and mental health. I try to offer support and kindness to my community of friends and family. And I try to be kind, polite and friendly to people I come in contact with throughout my day. I don't always succeed, but I do *try*. Almost every religion puts forth the idea that we should treat others as we wish to be treated. Even religions with very different belief systems agree upon *this*.

If I have a day wherein I'm not nice to someone, I find it difficult to be happy. Few of us take real pleasure in being unkind to another person. When it happens, it's usually because we're unhappy, or unsettled within ourselves.

If you want to stay youthful, happiness is certainly something you'll need to cultivate. Taking good care of your health, as I've suggested, will certainly help, but it's only a part of it. Practicing kindness towards others is a great way to cultivate deep happiness and that happiness will show up in your body, and spirit, and help keep you vibrant and young.

FINAL THOUGHTS

In closing, I'd like to emphasize that an approach to staying young doesn't have to cost a lot of money. If you follow the advice I've offered, you can avoid spending a fortune on plastic surgery and minor procedures, like Botox, or skin fillers, which, though not exorbitant in price, are not cheap, and add up over time. Habitually take excellent care of yourself and there will be no need to pay to fix the damage of improper care.

Another thing I should point out is that though what I've talked about may lead to beauty, good health (physical and mental) is the most important goal. Having beauty is lovely, but it should never be sought at the expense of health. And what *is* beauty, anyway? Though we may be able to define it, it's different for everyone. A more important goal is to simply be you—the best version of you.

Hope some of this has been helpful. I've so often been asked what the secret to my youthfulness is, and I wanted a way to share with people that it's not *one* thing, or even a few things-- it's *every*thing! It's a lifestyle, a mindset. It is a commitment to physical, mental, emotional, and spiritual health.

I wish you joy, health, love and beauty inside and out as you grow older. Life is so amazing. Enjoy every bit of it. Be happy and appreciate all that you are. Vibrate at the frequency of your very best self!

INTERVIEWS

The following section contains a series of interviews with several wise women in my life. They range in age from their 30s to their 60s, and each of them looks much younger than her actual age. They each had valuable secrets to share. I hope you'll benefit from them.

Apinya Pokachaiyapat

Born in Thailand Apinya came to the US to attend boarding school at age twelve. She holds degrees in mathematics, civil engineering, and creative writing. She is also a long-time Vipassana meditator, and Reiki practitioner. She received her Yoga teacher training from Yoga Works in Santa Monica, California. Her path has led her to many teachers and healers that have taught her various healing modalities. Her mentors include Jeanne Heileman, Annie Carpenter, and Birgitte Kristen. After years of training in the healing arts, in Apinya was inspired to open RakSa, an eco-friendly wellness center in Culver City, California.

What do you include in your diet to stay youthful and healthy?

Alkaline Water, mostly organic food: Kale, quinoa, Echinacea tea, and chocolate soy pudding (it's good for my soul).

What do you exclude from your diet to stay youthful and healthy?

Too much of any one thing, but mostly I avoid dairy, meat, and refined sugar.

What sort of exercise do you do?

Running, spinning, yoga, hiking, and walking on the beach. I did rock climbing for ten years, but not any more. Still, being outdoors will always make me truly happy.

How do you care for your skin?

I wash my face morning and night, then I use a toner and moisturizer with sunscreen for day and a lighter one for night (my favorite is Aveda Tourmaline Charged Protecting Lotion SPF 15/Oil Free). I exfoliate at least once a week both face and body. I get a monthly facial. I use a very simple and all natural body lotion, unscented. Epsom salt or tea bath for detoxifying.

Any beauty products you can't live without?

Jane Iredale Makeup (the most natural I've found).

Do you have a spiritual practice, and if so, do you think it's had any impact on your appearance?

Very much so. The inner peace reflects much greater than the outer appearance. I practice yoga daily, which for me, some days is just a 15 minute meditation. I study various ancient healings and spiritual fields. Writing is also my spiritual practice. Living in balance, or working on that balance-- getting closer to my true self, is my practice. Also when I am able to process my emotions and release them in a healthy way, my body doesn't hold onto it physically. Thus when I release what no longer serves me in the inside, the outside also falls away.

What were some challenges that led to your evolution?

Hormonal changes which affect my mood, my energy, and my distribution of weight.

If you were to advise a young woman on a few things you've learned about how to age well, what would those things be?

Listen to your body, it tells you exactly what you need or want to do; then actually do those. Accept yourself in all aspects. We all have limitations, but I don't think time is the main limitation to youth unless you let it be.

Any advice for older women on things they might do to turn back the clock?

Reevaluate you diet and eat more natural and things that are easier for your body to process, or that agree with your digestive system. Find a part of you that you may have neglected, or haven't been as in touch with, listen and get to know her. Do the things you've always wanted to do. Take some time for yourself everyday and breath deeply.

Dena Crowder

Dena is a success strategist and spiritual power guide. For 13 years, she's empowered people from all backgrounds and walks of life to awaken Heart and Soul. She brings her unique blend of universal principle and practical success techniques into the world of organizations through magical "team building" cooking experiences, conference keynotes, and customized retreats and seminars. Graduates of Dena's manifesting programs have published books, negotiated multi-million dollar deals, penned hit movies, and garnered numerous awards. *Dubbed "Hollywood's Success Coach" by the BBC and The Washington Post, a "Person to Watch" by the London Times, and declared a "Hot Topic" on Tv's The View, Dena has been featured in a variety of print media, including: The Seattle Times, The Los Angeles Independent, Essence magazine, The Washington Post, The Larchmont Chronicle, The Westchester County Business Journal, Body and Soul, The Aquarian Times, and DYSONNA magazine. She also hosted a weekly call in Success show on LA radio.* Dena graduated with honors from Marlborough School for Girls in Los Angeles, Columbia College in New York City, and she has a Master's degree from USC's School of Journalism. Personally trained by world renowned masters in human development, communication, success and spirituality, she is also a certified meditation teacher, energy expert, and a yogi.

What do you include in your diet to stay youthful and healthy?

First thing after waking up, I put a kettle of water on. When the water is nearly boiling, I pour enough hot water into a heat-proof glass to create a half and half combination of hot water to room temperature water. I add a generous squeeze of lemon, and drink. This hydrates the body, wakes up your digestion, and encourages your body's natural release process. (Some people have a bowel movement soon after doing this.) Next, a fresh juice of kale, apple, cucumber, and orange. Cucumber is very anti-aging according to nutritionists, and the benefits of the other ingredients are self-evident.

*I don't allow myself to have coffee or my beloved darjeeling tea until I've done at least one, and most of the time, both processes above. *

I also include lots of vitamin C in food based or crystal form.

What do you exclude from your diet to stay youthful and healthy?

In general, I exclude sodas, deep fried foods, packaged sugary and salty snacks (like potato chips, Doritos, etc) and mainstream fast food. I do, however give myself an occasional treat. If I have a tremendous day, or a wonderful accomplishment occurs, I reward myself with a Coke on ice and a lime twist. While this is a "special" moment, I mention it because I've seen many people shut down joy and *life happening* as they attempt to rigidly practice healthy eating. I believe that if a food/meal brings you joy, even if its fried chicken and a coke, then it can have a spiritual, and thus revitalizing affect. As long as you are following a healthy diet most of the time, the occasional indulgence--a slice of cake at a dear friend's wedding, you grandmother's famous ribs on her 90th birthday—is fine.

What sort of exercise to you do?

YOGA: Hatha and Kundalini, Basic Chi Gong

How do you care for your skin?

For my Face: I use a natural skin care line created by a healer named Barbara Rogers. She energizes her products with Reikki, and they feel very alive as they penetrate into the skin. (Simply Divine Botanicals) They can be ordered through the Internet.

I find its important to switch cleansers, so your skin doesn't get lazy. I supplement the Simply Divine face wash with a gorgeous handmade soap by an African-American woman owned company named Kaeli's. The owner, Kaeli, used to have a store in my neighborhood, and her black soap, called Tribal Mud, is incredible. Don't quote me, but I believe it has 32 ayuervedic herbs/ingredients. She can also be found on the Internet. (Kaelibodycare.com)

Do you have a spiritual practice and if so, do you think it's had any impact on your appearance?

Yes. A daily spiritual practice can reverse the aging process. Literally. I have meditated daily for 14 years. My meditation practice is the single most potent factor, in my opinion, that contributes to my youthful appearance and my vitality. A rich spiritual practice gives us an inner radiance. It also youthens the physical organs, keeps the brain alert, and relieves stress, and can prevent disease.

What were some challenges that led to your evolution?

Life challenges can put the years and lines on your face, or they can liberate you into more radiance. I have chosen the latter. We all face obstacles and experience pain. We can choose whether to "carry" the pain or to allow something deeper to express through us.

In my own life, I've faced financial challenges (starting a business no one understood, or thought would succeed in an era before life coaching/yoga was a household word) and health challenges (my spiritual path began with an illness). When we're in the midst of uncomfortable circumstances, our tendency is to think about all the negative potential outcomes, and to desperately search for a way to fix what we believe is wrong. This keeps us in a loop. A more empowering approach is to practice mindfulness, that is, clearing the mind of the negative chatter, allowing ourselves to find a place of peace even in the middle of our trials and tribulations. In this way, we release carrying the weight (of fear and negativity), we relax into peace, and are then open to ask deeper questions, like: "what is trying to express through me now? What is my soul's vision of this situation? How can I embody my soul's vision through this situation? What is this seeming problem gifting me?"

If you were to advise a young woman on a few things you've learned about how to age well, what would those things be?

Practice forgiveness. Forgiveness is a powerful anti-aging secret. To forgive means to move beyond a place we've been stuck. If we've been holding a grudge against someone, to forgive them doesn't mean we sanction their actions: it simply means we stop dragging them and our hurt/anger around. We let go. We move on. Anger, fear, hatred, bitterness, and the culture of complaint make abysmal cosmetics. The willingness to forgive frees up stuck energy, releases radiance, brightens our skin and improves our total quality of life.

Have you noticed that women who are holding onto things age very poorly? People say: "wow, she looks hard." Or "Father Time's beat her with an old stick," as they notice how devoid of life force and vitality they are.

Forgiveness works as a magical salve way beyond the beauty quest. If an area of your life is really stuck, chances are there is something you'd do well to forgive in that area.

Love yourself unreservedly. That comes first. Without self-love, we look to fill a void with external stimuli, be it food, alcohol, too many late nights, excess shopping, or the lover who's wrong for you. Without self-love, we seek to "fill up" our tank from the outside--resulting in an incessant quest to get (status, money, recognition, you name it). In the end, you'll come across as desperate and age badly. As women age, character comes forward, and is a greater factor in the perception of beauty. Participate actively in service.   Give to someone else. Care for others. Remember how beautiful Audrey Hepburn looked in her later years as a good will ambassador? That's the power of service.

Any advice for older women on thing they might do to turn back the clock?

Meditate and exercise! Go ahead. Start now.

Anja Lee

Anja is a traveler at heart. Born in Canada, she grew up in Connecticut, went to college in the Midwest and lived in England and Holland. She eventually made her way back via a circular route to her true home in New York City. She still hasn't decided what she will be when she grows up (and that may never happen), but for now she enjoys being an actress, singer, writer, model, teacher, trainer, and real estate investor. Her passion is world travel, having visited over 60 countries and still counting. Anja found a natural and healthy lifestyle a few years ago and has never looked back. She is happy to have discovered that youth, beauty and health are maintained as much through what we put "in" our bodies as it is by what we put "on" them.

What do you include in your diet to stay youthful and healthy?

I include 100 percent whole grain breads, cage free organic free range eggs with omega 3s, brown rice, green tea, leafy greens, blueberries, spinach, dark chocolate, tons of fruits, and lots and lots of water.

What do you exclude from your diet to stay youthful and healthy?

I read labels on food religiously. If it has more than 5 ingredients it's too processed. If it has anything I can't pronounce or don't recognize it is probably a chemical additive. I avoid added sugar, high fructose corn syrup, and any type of hydrogenated oil. I avoid white rice, white flour products, and products with wheat gluten. Instead I use whole grain products (they have to say 100 percent whole grain or they aren't) brown rice pasta, gluten free breads and cereals. I avoid yogurt with flavors as they have sugar added and prefer plain, organic yogurt where I can add my own fruit and maybe some agave syrup.

What sort of exercise do you do?

I work out with a personal trainer once a week to push myself, and our workouts include a full core workout. Even if we are working legs, we are also working core. She is a Pilates instructor, yoga instructor, Capoeira (Brazilian martial arts) instructor, and a massage therapist; so the workouts are varied and interesting and target every part of the body. It is also important to do more that one thing at a time to challenge the body and the brain. For instance, don't just do stationary curls for the arms with weights. Why not challenge the core by standing on a Bosu (a core strength stability ball) while doing this, or try standing on one leg as you do the exercise. This will force you to contact your core to balance, and it will force you to concentrate on the workout. My workouts don't allow for sitting on the bike and reading a book. They should challenge me more than that. When I'm not with the trainer, I like a combo of cardio on the elliptical, yoga, Pilates, weight training, etc. Variety is the key to keep from being bored and to keep the body from getting used to the same old exercise routine and hitting a plateau. Blood sugar levels fluctuate after workouts, so be sure to have a healthy snack before and after exercising, like an apple and a few almonds.

How do you care for your skin?

I use all natural skin care products. When I stopped eating chemicals and cleaning my house with chemicals, I also started buying all natural skincare products. I like the EO (essential oils) brand of bodywashes and lotions, because they're filled with antioxidants for skin. Exfoliation is key and I like Derma e Microdermabrasion scrub for home use. My skin always glows after this. I also like products with 10 percent glycolic acid to remove dead skin cells and make the skin glow. I like an all natural sea salt or sugar body scrub to exfoliate the body. There is a spa called Elina Skin Care in Michigan that makes all of their own all-natural products and I have found them very helpful to combat acne naturally. All of their products are filled with vitamins, minerals, and antioxidants and are affordable compared to department store beauty products.

Do you have a spiritual practice, and if so, do you think it's had any impact on your appearance?

Yoga is a spiritual practice for me. I spent a month at a yoga resort/ retreat a few years back, and I left feeling better than I ever have. I felt slim and happy with my body for the first time I could remember. I left relaxed, feeling and looking very young.

Traveling is also a spiritual experience for me. The importance of vacationing, visiting new places, experiencing new things should not be over looked. Vacations are as important to me as paying rent, and I do my best to make sure I take a few weeks every year. Even if I am short on money, I may take a shorter one or research budget locations where the dollar will stretch, but I always take a vacation, because I need it to relax, and feed my soul. This year I went to Bali, which is a beautiful spiritual place and though it is a long journey there, it is incredibly inexpensive when you get there. There are still places in the world where our dollar can go far!

Every year after my vacation I feel and look refreshed, renewed, and ready to tackle the urban jungle of NYC that I call home.

What were some challenges that resulted in your evolution?

Back in 2006 I attended a health seminar at a wonderful place called the Kripalu Center in the Berkshires, MA. I had been battling several different health issues, none life threatening, but they were definitely burdening me. I had no health insurance so it was costing me a fortune out of pocket, and I was relatively young and healthy, but taking 6 different prescriptions, each for a symptom, yet no one could tell me what the root of this problem was. I was at my wits end, disgusted with modern medicine, and needing relief. This health seminar was lead by Dr. Mark Hyman and he changed my life. Kripalu has become my spiritual and health mecca. Dr. Hyman and his associates have become my Doctors, and I transitioned to an all-natural lifestyle, and even got off the 6 prescriptions I was taking. My thyroid medication is the only one I still take, but the other symptoms were cleared up with the use of supplements and changing my diet.

If you were to advise a young woman on a few things you've learned about how to age well, what would those things be?

For young women I would say don't get complacent and think that you don't have to worry about aging until you get older. You will wake up one day and realize it has caught up to you, so better to take care of your skin, health, weight etc. now so that you don't have regrets. You can make beneficial changes at any age, but the younger you start the more success you will have. Exfoliate!!! Get enough sleep. Vitamins. Exercise. Minimize junk food. Sunscreen. And nourishing moisturizers!

Any advice for older women on things they might do to turn back the clock?

For older women, it is never too late to incorporate change in to your life style. My mother now uses a personal trainer, and though she is 68 and cannot fully turn back the hands of time, she went from a sedentary lifestyle to one where she can lift more weights than I can. No joke. So Exercise, eat right, be good to your body and your mind. Delight in life and you. Care for your skin. You will see results.
www.anjalee.net

Angela de Joseph

Angela de Joseph started her career as the associate beauty editor at Essence Magazine. She went on to be the creative director of Johnson Products Company, and the founding editor of Sophisticate's Black Hair Styles and Care Guide. Since then she became the on-camera fashion and beauty expert on "Live With Regis and Kathie," and "AM Los Angeles." She went on to serve as a spokesperson for clients such as Dupont Fibers, JC Penny and Woolite, logging over 300 television appearances in the top 20 media markets. Enrolling in film school was a major turning point in Angela's life. She wrote, produced and directed an award-winning film, entitled, "It's In The Bag," which was showcased on Showtime and BET networks. Utilizing her filmmaking skills, and drawing on her experience as a beauty editor, and daughter of a beauty entrepreneur, Angela created African Wonders Hair Products and developed a multi-million dollar television infomercial. Today, Angela has embraced her passion for health and fitness and is the author of, "The Body-Blast: Heal Your Soul and Your Body Will Follow," a motivational book chronicling her challenges and triumph over her own weight issues. She served as Director of Arise Health Center a community based health advocacy program in Westchester, California. Through this program she taught nutrition classes, and produced health fairs and weight-loss clinics. This year

Angela is launching BeautyWellnessTV.com a web portal for health and beauty which features her own web series, "The Angela de Joseph Show."
http://www.theAngeladeJosephShow.com

What do you include in your diet to stay youthful and healthy?

I add living foods to my diet. Raw plant foods have enzymes that detoxify and nourish the body on a cellular level. The more fresh organic fruit and vegetables I eat the better I look and feel.

What do you exclude from your diet to stay youthful and healthy?

I do not eat red meat or poultry. The food chain is poisoned with antibiotics, steroids, hormones, and diseased animals recycled as feed.

What sort of exercise to you do?

My exercise routine includes cardio, resistance training, yoga and pilates. I work out 5 days a week. I start with a half hour of power walking or jogging then do a half hour of weight lifting and end with pilates core exercises and a yoga stretching routine.

How do you care for your skin?

I use a gentle exfoliating cleanser, followed by a moisturizer with a sunscreen daily.

Any beauty products you can't live without?

I love eyeliner. If I have eyeliner on I'm made up. It defines my eyes and makes me feel attractive.

Do you have a spiritual practice, and if so, do you think it's had any impact on your appearance?

I am a Christian and I read a book called "Handbook To Prayer: Praying Scripture Back To God," each morning. It settles my spirit and gives me comfort, which translates to a better mind set all day.

What were some challenges that resulted in your evolution?

I am a product of an immigrant West Indian family. Trying to assimilate into the American culture caused friction in our lives. My parents were divorced when I was child. I found comfort in food and struggled with weight and self-esteem issues throughout my life. Being saved and developing a closer walk with God has filled the emotional hole in my soul, and allowed me to claim the victory over childhood pain. I have to continually replenish through reading the Bible and staying close to uplifting, like-minded people.

If you were to advise a young woman on a few things you've learned about how to age well, what would those things be?

You are your most valuable asset. Treat yourself with the care you would give to a Rolls Royce. You wouldn't put cheap gas in a Rolls Royce, so don't put junk food into your body. You wouldn't drive around in a dirty Rolls Royce, so don't leave the house looking like a mess. You wouldn't let a person you don't know, or an irresponsible person drive your Rolls Royce, so don't let anyone who isn't worthy, take you for a spin.

Any advice for older women on thing they might do to turn back the clock?

There are two areas that age, your body and your brain. To reverse the aging of your body, eat fresh organic fruit and vegetables daily and exercise 5-6 days a week. To reverse the aging of your brain spend time with youthful, fun people.

Anything else you'd like to share?

Everyone looks and feels better when they have love. Find someone to love and let someone love you.

Candace Wilson Culp

At 17 years old, a week after graduating high school Candace was hired to work at the Sands Hotel in Las Vegas as one of the "World famous Copa Girls." She was thrown into a world where appearance and presence was all. From there she went to New York to become a model, while she supported herself at night as a showgirl/dancer at the Latin Quarter and the Copacabana. She continued modeling while living in Europe for 2 years before returning to Los Angeles where she lived for 38 years. She married, divorced, went to UCLA design school, remarried (actor Robert Culp) and then became a mother at 33. Candace focused on being "just a mom," as her daughter liked to characterize her throughout her childhood. She began designing jewelry at her dining room table and then when her daughter was 16, she began dealing in antiques and taking on interior design clients.

What do you include in your diet to stay youthful and healthy?

When I was a young model I was focused on the need to stay so thin for so for many years that I know I shorted my body on what it needed. Now I try to remember to nurture myself with things we now know are so important like salmon and berries and high protein, complex carbohydrates like quinoa. I have always loved all vegetables. My weaknesses are chocolate, ice cream, and I love to drink red wine! Also I try to make sure to take my vitamins; Optivite, they're great and really do make a difference in my energy level.

What do you exclude from your diet to stay youthful and healthy?

I try to watch my white carbs and I am trying to become a vegetarian for moral reasons, though I know it would have far reaching health benefits.

What sort of exercise do you do?

I love walking in cities where there is much to look at, and I loved beginning ballet classes, but I have never liked traditional sports or exercise much until I discovered The Lotte Berk Method, and later Pilates. They both stretch your muscles and make you strong. Recently we got a home version Pilates machine, so I am going to begin again, now, to get back in shape. I don't believe it's too late.

How do you care for your skin?

I was never in the sun much; It was too boring to lay in the sun for hours and then as a model in the late 60s a tan was verboten. I began using Retin-A about 20 years ago and I really believe it contributed to having a complexion that may be a little younger than my age. I have really dry skin so I have always used a lot of lotion after a bath...Lubriderm was a staple and now Eucerin. Also I have used the same hand lotion since I was 6 years old, Aquamarine by Revlon...I don't know if it does anything but it smells divine.

My only absolute is that I don't go to bed without removing my makeup. I cleanse using Cetaphil Lotion, or Clarins Sensitive Skin Cream Cleanser. I have always used a makeup foundation and I remember a dermatologist once saying that was a good idea since we know the ingredients of the makeup but not what's in the air...she felt it acted as a shield. At any rate, I think it protected from the sun even before we became aware of the need for sunscreen. Later I became a fanatic about using a moisturizer with a good SPF. Neutrogena Healthy Face works well for me.

Any beauty products you can't live without?

Moisturizer, hand lotion, and lipstick (the new Revlon one that stays on it just great!) I never spend a moment without it. Eye shadow and eye pencil are pretty much everyday necessities also. I've recently stopped using mascara and I think it looks more natural for me.

Do you have a spiritual practice and if so, do you think it's had any impact on your appearance?

I believe that when you give to other people and feel the joy that you receive in return it does something special for your appearance…I admire people who have a spiritual practice in the conventional sense, but I am a bit undisciplined. My goal this year is to meditate on a daily basis, as I believe it can change how you perceive your reality.

What were some challenges that resulted in your evolution?

Wow, this is a difficult one, I can only hope I have evolved some…I think I have always been lucky in terms of my health until a few years a few years ago. To know what it's like to go to bed in pain and wake up in pain and spend the day in pain was a real revelation. I wish I had learned that sooner. I like to believe that I would have been kinder and more patient with many people in my life.

If you were to advise a young woman on a few things you've learned about how to age well, what would those things be?

Having spent so much of my life in the business of beauty I learned very late what was really important. I think to contribute more to other beings is the real way to age well. This was late coming, but is my work in progress.

Any advice for older women on things they might do to turn back the clock?

I think I look my best when I am excited about something. Find something you are passionate about…that is a real age eraser. Think of how beautiful Jane Goodall is after a lifetime spent in Africa.

Anything else you'd like to share?

I was recently looking at old photos and was amazed at how good I looked, yet then I could only see what was lacking. I will never be that age and state again, too bad I didn't appreciate it then. A few months ago I took a silly fall and went flying across the room and crashed my head into the bathroom counter resulting in a dreadful cut across above one eyebrow requiring 7 stitches, luckily just missing my eye. That kind of thing, having a big scar, losing control over my appearance would have devastated me as recently as ten years ago. I am amazed at my change in attitude, I even kind of like my scar. Perhaps perfect is no longer perfect!

CITATIONS

I've included links that cover the topics I discuss in the text. You can use them for further research.

*note: The dates listed are the date on which the links were retrieved.

Chapter: Returning the Body to its Purest State and Maintaining it

Master Cleanse
http://themastercleanse.org/
April 22, 2010

Mucoid Plaque myth
· _ab_"Mucoid Plaque". Quackwatch.
http://www.quackwatch.org/04ConsumerEducation/QA/mucoidplaque.html.

_ab_"Ed's Guide to Alternative Therapies: Colonics".
April 21, 2010

Lining of the colon same as the lining of the mouth
http://www.pathguy.com/altermed.htm#colonic.
April 21, 2010

Benefits of dietary fiber
http://www.carbs-information.com/dietary-fiber-benefits.htm
April 21, 2010

How fiber rich foods cleanse the colon
http://ezinearticles.com/?High-Fiber-Foods----How-Does-Fiber-Rich-Foods-Help-in-Colon--Cleansing?&id=1932106>.
April 22, 2010

Exfoliating is regenerative
http://www.ehow.com/about_6196813_meaning-exfoliate_.html
April 21, 2010

Dental Plaque
http://www.healingdaily.com/conditions/bleeding-gums.htm
April 21, 2010

Periodontal disease and Alzheimer's disease
http://www.colgate.com/app/Colgate/US/OC/Information/ADA/Article_2005_09_ADAAlzheimers.cvsp
April 22, 2010

Benefits of flossing on the Brain
http://indianapublicmedia.org/amomentofscience/mental-dental/

April 25, 2010

Dental Plaque and Heart health
http://www.perio.org/consumer/plaque-risk.htm
April 25, 2010

Bacteria under the nails
http://shine.yahoo.com/channel/health/5-frightening-truths-about-the-germs-under-your-fingernails-and-his-332777/
April 22, 2010

Chapter: Brush Your Face

Exfoliating brings oxygen to the skin
https://secure.earthsaversonline.com/earthsavers_lifestyle_tip_details.php?tip_category_id=5&tip_id=23
April 22, 2010

Chapter: Take Omega 3's

Dr. Perricone and Omega 3s
http://en.wikipedia.org/wiki/Nicholas_Perricone
August 22, 2010

Benefit's of Omega 3;s
http://ezinearticles.com/?3-Skin-Care-Benefits-From-Taking-Omega-3-Fish-Oil-Supplements&id=2355794

August 14, 2010

Chapter: Take a Multivitamin

Benefits of taking a multivitamin
http://ezinearticles.com/?The-Benefits-of-Taking-a-Daily-Multivitamin&id=79596
April 22, 2010

Anti-Aging benefits of multivitamins
http://EzineArticles.com/?expert=Cynthia_Wang-Tan
April 22, 2010

Vitamins improve looks
http://www.freearticles.com/article/Vitamins-Improve-Appearance/2851
April 22, 2010

Dr. Oz recommends multivitamins
http://www.oprah.com/health/Dr-Ozs-Ultimate-Anti-Aging-Checklist/19
April 22, 2010

Vitamins and what they do:
http://www.buzzle.com/articles/vitamins-and-what-they-do.html
April 22, 2010

Vitamin A's benefit to skin:
http://www.womens-health-questions.com/vitamin-a-skin-care.html

April 22, 2010

Vitamin A enhances the skin:
http://healing.about.com/od/acne/a/acnevita
mins.htm
April 22, 2010

Chapter: Eat Gelatin

Collagen and firmer skin:
http://www.oprah.com/style/Beauty-Around-
the-World/2
August 11, 2011

http://www.jstage.jst.go.jp/article/jnsv/52/3/
52_211/_article
August 11, 2011

Chapter: Drink Aloe Vera Juice

Benefits of Aloe Vera Juice
http://www.americanchronicle.com/articles/vi
ew/29154
August 14, 2010

"Effect of Orally consumed Aloe Vera Juice," by
Jeffrey Bland, Ph.D.
http://asktom-
naturally.com/naturally/aloevera.html
August 14, 2010

Using Aloe Vera externally to benefit the skin

http://www.ehow.com/how_2330460_treat-facial-wrinkles-aloe-vera.html
August 14, 2010

http://www.beautyandgroomingtips.com/2006/06/aloevera-wonder-herb.html
August 14, 2010

Chapter: Apple Cider Vinegar

Information on ACV
http://www.webmd.com/diet/apple-cider-vinegar
August 14, 2010

http://altmedicine.about.com/od/applecidervinegardiet/a/applecidervineg_2.htm
August 14, 2010

http://ezinearticles.com/?Apple-Cider-Vinegar---The-Miracle-That-Makes-You-Ageless&id=1431107
August 14, 2010

Chapter: Coconut Oil

Fife, Bruce. <u>The Coconut Oil Miracle.</u> Penguin Group: New York, 2004.

Chemicals absorbed by the skin
http://www.osha.gov/SLTC/dermalexposure/index.html

August 14, 2010

Chapter: Olive Oil

Olive oil benefits
http://www.thedailygreen.com/green-homes/latest/olive-oil-benefits-uses-460609
August 4, 2010

http://www.naturalskincaresecrets.com/olive-oil-skin-care.html
August 15, 2010

Chapter: Neem Oil

Neem oil's benefit to skin
http://www.discoverneem.com/neem-oil-for-skin.html
August 4, 2010

Chapter: Shea Butter

http://www.vitaminstuff.com/supplements-shea-butter.html
August 15, 2010

Benefits of Shea Butter
http://www.ehow.com/facts_4796989_dermatological-benefits-shea-butter.html
August 15, 2010

Cinnamic acid

http://www.ncbi.nlm.nih.gov/pubmed/184515
24
August 15, 2010

Chapter: Fasting

Mucoid Plaque myth
http://en.wikipedia.org/wiki/Mucoid_plaque
August 16, 2010

Layers of intestinal wall
http://informahealthcare.com/doi/abs/10.3109
/00365528609091857
August 16, 2010

Master Cleanse
http://en.wikipedia.org/wiki/Master_Cleanse
August 16, 2010

A body that's pure
http://www.projo.com/health/content/lb_deto
x_02-04-07_IB3JLKK.50def6d.html
August 16, 2010

Chapter: Drink Only Liquids that Provide Nutrition, Cleanse or Hydrate

Soda and Osteoporosis
http://www.webmd.com/osteoporosis/feature
s/soda-osteoporosis
August 16, 2010

Dangers of high fructose corn syrup
http://www.princeton.edu/main/news/archiv
e/S26/91/22K07/
August 16, 2010

Coffee has antioxidants
http://www.physorg.com/news6067.html
August 16, 2010

Green tea
http://www.oprah.com/style/Dr-Perricones-
Prescription-for-Aging-Beautifully
August 16, 2010

Green tea fights wrinkles and aids weight loss
http://shine.yahoo.com/event/green/nine-
reasons-to-drink-green-tea-daily-1609132/
June 11, 2010

Red wine benefits
http://www.mayoclinic.com/health/red-
wine/hb00089
April 23, 2010

Revesveratrol and bone density

http://docs.google.com/viewer?a=v&q=cache:i
yCNmhm7XD8J:ijbs.org/User/ContentFullText.
aspx%3FVolumeNO%3D1%26StartPage%3D76%
26Type%3Dpdf+resveratrol+and+bone+density
&hl=en&gl=us&pid=bl&srcid=ADGEESjEbN3V
wck8T0ZHruuI1m8IS1jgA92Sk3h20XXljPBpZ9t
U6rxoFZdf4uFCSCjSkwpC572DHGJgskvoRaCQ
OdHkR1WZK1MYLomQlm4TzIzmk1cONJtL1F
gl5yTHYFMu49vTQb2E&sig=AHIEtbRBjBXU_Z
4RG1bjFM3vcGgJ2sQSwQ
April 23, 2010

Red wine and bone density
http://lifestyle.iloveindia.com/lounge/health-
benefits-of-red-wine-8758.html
April 23, 2010

Alcohol dehydrates the body
http://www.islamawareness.net/Alcohol/alco
hol_news_007.html
August 16, 2010

Sugar is aging
http://www.cnet.com/8301-13553_1-9811304-
32.html
August 16, 2010

How sugar makes us age
http://longevity.about.com/od/researchandme
dicine/p/crosslinking.htm
August 16, 2010

Dangers of sugar substitutes
http://www.womentowomen.com/healthywei
ght/splenda.aspx
August 16, 2010

Honey has antioxidants
Science news July 18, 1998
http://www.sciencedaily.com/releases/1998/0
7/980708085352.htm
April 23, 2010

More on honey
.
http://www.nal.usda.gov/fnic/foodcomp/sear
ch/
· ^ a b ([dead link]) Questions Most Frequently
Asked About Sugar. American Sugar Alliance.
http://www.sugaralliance.org/desktopdefault.a
spx?page_id=97.
· ^ Martos I, Ferreres F, Tomás-Barberán F
(2000). "Identification of flavonoid markers for
the botanical origin of Eucalyptus honey". *J Agric
Food Chem* **48** (5): 1498–502.
doi:10.1021/jf991166q. PMID 10820049.

Maple syrup contains calcium and iron,
magnesium and potassium and Omega6 fatty
acids
http://www.nutritiondata.com/facts/sweets/5
602/2
April 23, 2010

Molasses contains health benefits
http://www.ehow.com/facts_4809658_health-benefits-molasses.html
May 2, 2010

Chapter: Eat Only (or at least mostly) Foods That Have Nutritional Value

Medicinal benefits of whole foods
http://www.moonsmuses.com/health.html
August 17, 2010

The effect of carbohydrates on blood sugar
http://www.hsph.harvard.edu/nutritionsource/what-should-you-eat/carbohydrates-full-story/index.html
August 17, 2010

Health benefits of Nuts
http://www.medicinenet.com/script/main/art.asp?articlekey=56560
August 17, 2010

Dangers of too much soy in the diet
http://www.scientificamerican.com/article.cfm?id=soybean-fertility-hormone-isoflavones-genistein
August 17, 2010

Dangers of processed meats

http://www.reuters.com/article/idUSTRE64G5
TN20100517
August 17, 2010

Chapter: Raw Foods

Raw food diet
http://altmedicine.about.com/od/popularhealt
hdiets/a/Raw_Food.htm
August 17, 2010

Chapter: Eat a Variety of Colors

Colors in foods and the benefits
http://www.buildingbodies.ca/Nutrition/fruits
-vegetables.shtml
August 17, 2010

Super foods
http://www.webmd.com/diet/guide/10-
everyday-super-foods?page=2
August 17, 2010

Chapter: Avoid Too Many Plastic Containers

Don't eat foods microwaved in plastics
http://shine.yahoo.com/event/loveyourbody/
why-you-cant-lose-those-last-10-pounds-
1964849/
July 20, 2010

Chapter: Avoid Too Much Alcohol

Alcohol and the Brain
http://ezinearticles.com/?Alcohol-Addiction-and-Brain-Adaptation---The-Long-Term-Impact-on-the-Brain&id=3438630
August 17, 2010

Alcohol's negative effects on the body
http://findarticles.com/p/articles/mi_m0847/is_n4_v13/ai_8276626/
August 17, 2010

Chapter: NOOOOOO Smoking!

Smoking ages you
http://www.ivillage.co.uk/beauty/skincare/aging/articles/0,,547681_613918,00.html
August 17, 2010

Chapter: Remove your Makeup and Wash and Moisturize Your Face Every Night

Reasons to wash your face at night
http://www.temptalia.com/skincare-tips-5-reasons-to-wash-your-face-at-night
August 17, 2010

Moisturize your skin while you sleep
http://www.articlesbase.com/skin-care-articles/moisture-skinnight-moisturizer-while-you-sleep-2158307.html
August 17, 2010

Chapter: Wide-brimmed Hats and Sunscreen

Aging and the sun
http://www.skincarephysicians.com/agingskin
net/basicfacts.html
August 17, 2010

Effects of the sun on skin
http://dermatology.about.com/cs/beauty/a/s
uneffect.htm
August 17, 2010

Our need for Vitamin D from the sun
http://health.usnews.com/health-news/family-
health/heart/articles/2008/06/23/time-in-the-
sun-how-much-is-needed-for-vitamin-d.html
August 17, 2010

Lycopene helps protect skin from the sun
http://naturalskinhealth.com/blog/skin-sun-
damage/
August 17, 2010

Chapter: Brushing, Flossing and Peroxide

Flossing can add years to your life and keep
arteries young
http://www.21stcenturydental.com/smith/edu
cation/floss.htm
August 19, 2010

Peroxide and teeth whitening
http://hubpages.com/hub/Hydrogen-
Peroxide-Teeth-Whitening
August 19, 2010

Chapter: Walk, Walk, Walk, Weights, Water

Exercise slows aging
http://www.washingtonpost.com/wp-
dyn/content/article/2008/01/28/AR200801280
1873.html
June 1, 2010

The effects of exercise on the brain
http://serendip.brynmawr.edu/bb/neuro/neur
o05/web2/mmcgovern.html
August 30, 2010

Cardio vs. Strength training
http://www.womenshealthmag.com/fitness/ca
rdio-vs-strength-training-workouts
August 30, 2010

Building muscle is better than cardio alone
http://strengthtraining.suite101.com/article.cf
m/why_building_muscle_is_better_than_cardio
_alone
August 30, 2010

Strength training helps the bones retain calcium
http://www.naturalnews.com/010528.html
August 30, 2010

Drinking water helps to burn fat
http://findarticles.com/p/articles/mi_m0KFY/
is_11_26/ai_n31144415
August 30, 2010

Chapter: Stair climbing

Benefits of stair climbing
http://www.nytimes.com/2009/02/19/health/
nutrition/19fitness.html
August 11, 2011

http://www.nytimes.com/2011/03/11/health/
nutrition/11urbathlete.html
August 11, 2011
http://www.hr.duke.edu/benefits/wellness/ex
ercise/stairwell/benefits.php

Stair climbing and improved bone density
http://www.osteopenia3.com/bone-density-
exercises.html
August 11, 2011

Chapter: Stretch

Stretching is anti-aging
http://www.streetdirectory.com/travel_guide/
23003/fitness/stretching_exercises_help_grow__
muscles__anti_aging_benefits.html
August 30, 2010

http://lifetwo.com/production/node/20071016
-aging-backwards-tuesday-tips-18-its-a-stretch
August 30, 2010

Chapter: Massage

"5 Surprising Benefits of Massage"
http://www.newsweek.com/2008/09/03/five-
surprising-benefits-of-massage.html
August 30, 2010

Chapter: Sleep

How sleep affects the aging process
http://www.immortalhumans.com/how-sleep-
effects-your-longevity-slumber-habits-impact-
life-extension/
August 30, 2010

Sleep and youthfulness
http://www.medicinenet.com/script/main/art.
asp?articlekey=54286
August 30, 2010

Chapter: Careful HOW You Sleep

Sleep on your back
http://www.webmd.com/skin-
beauty/features/23-ways-to-reduce-wrinkles
August 30, 2010

Chapter: Sex

Having sex frequently can make you look up to 12 years younger
http://www.prevention.com/8easyageerasers/list/2.shtml
August 31, 2010

Orgasm is a stress reliever
http://www.todaysmodernfamily.com/index.php/tag/orgasm-is-a-stress-reliever
August 31 2010

Benefits of orgasm
http://www.livestrong.com/article/13903-orgasm-benefits/
August 31, 2010

10 benefits of sex
http://www.webmd.com/sex-relationships/features/10-surprising-health-benefits-of-sex?page=3
August 31, 2010

Chapter: Clearing Old emotions — Cry It Out

Healing emotional wounds
http://www.ehow.com/how_4558328_heal-emotional-wounds-scars.html
August 31, 2010

How to forgive

http://stress.about.com/od/relationships/a/how_to_forgive.htm
August 31, 2010

Chapter: Clear Old Junk From Your Living Space

Benefits of getting rid of clutter
http://home-organization.suite101.com/article.cfm/10_great_reasons_to_get_rid_of_clutter
August 31, 2010

Well-being comes from getting rid of old stuff
http://fengshui.about.com/od/thebasics/qt/clearclutter.htm
August 31, 2010

Chapter: Add Some Life To Your Living Space

Benefits of indoor plants
http://www.buzzle.com/articles/benefits-of-indoor-plants.html
September 1, 2010

The effect of color
http://iit.bloomu.edu/vthc/design/psychology.htm
September 1, 2010

Chapter: Get Out in Nature

Benefits of trees
http://www.growingplanet.org/benefitoftrees.
html
September 1, 2010

Psychological benefits of green space
http://www.ncbi.nlm.nih.gov/pmc/articles/P
MC2390667/
September 1, 2010

Chapter: Non-Toxic Cleaning

Dr. Oz recommended non-toxic cleaner
http://www.adventuresofaglutenfreemom.com
/2010/04/homemade-safe-cleanser-recipe-from-
the-dr-oz-show/
September 1, 2010

Chapter: Non-Toxic Gardening

Vinegar as a weed killer
http://landscaping.about.com/od/weedsdiseas
es/qt/vinegar_weeds.htm
September 2, 2010

What is a watershed and how it affects
communities
http://www.watershedatlas.org/fs_indexwater.
html
September 2, 2010

Benefits of composting
http://www.denvergov.com/OrganicsProgram
s/CompostingCollectionPilotProgram/Benefitso
fComposting/tabid/433350/Default.aspx
September 2, 2010

Chapter: Potions for those over 45: hyrdroquinone, Minoxidil, dye

Benefits and risks of hydroquinone
http://www.smartskincare.com/conditions/pig
mentation/hyperpigmentation-treatments.html
September 2, 2010

Benefits and risks of Minoxidil
http://www.drugs.com/cons/minoxidil-
topical.html
September 2, 2010

To dye or not to dye
http://www.time.com/time/nation/article/0,8
599,1658058-2,00.html
September 2, 2010

Risks of permanent hair dye
http://www.fitgroove.com/hair/risks-of-
dying-hair.asp
September 2, 2010

Chapter: Meditation/Prayer

Meditate to maintain youth

http://www.ehow.com/how_2134253_maintain
-youth-intelligence.html
September 3, 2010

Meditation can help you look younger
http://ezinearticles.com/?Meditation-Can-
Help-You-Look-Younger&id=3348229
September 3, 2010

Chapter: Visualization

Why visualization works
http://behavioural-
psychology.suite101.com/article.cfm/visualizati
on
September 3, 2010

Chapter: Optimism

Benefits of Optimism
http://www.maxmore.com/optimism.htm
September 3, 2010

Chapter: Gratitude

Health benefits of almonds
http://www.cfidsselfhelp.org/library/counting
-your-blessings-how-gratitude-improves-your-
health
September 3, 2010

Chapter: Don't focus your energy on changing others

The futility of trying to control others
http://www.askdanandjennifer.com/love-relationships/relationship-advice/the-hidden-dangers-of-trying-to-control-your-husband-or-wife/
September 3, 2010

Chapter: Learn Something New

How the brain benefits from learning new things
http://www.bhia.org/articles/aging/learningtostayyoung.html
September 3, 2010

Chapter: Be Good to Others

Happiness
http://www.happinessinthisworld.com/2010/08/15/when-you-dont-like-yourself/?sms_ss=facebook
September 4, 2010

TONI ANN JOHNSON received a BFA from New York University's Tisch School of the Arts and an MFA in Creative Writing from Antioch University. An award-winning screenwriter, she won a fellowship to the Sundance Institute's Screenwriting Lab. She also won The Christopher Award and The Humanitas Prize for her teleplay, "Ruby Bridges," (ABC). She won The Humanitas Prize again for her teleplay, "Crown Heights," (Showtime). Also a playwright, her work has been produced by The Negro Ensemble Company and by The New York Stage and Film Company. Toni Ann also writes about community beautification in South Los Angeles and about health and beauty. She blogs at www.Vibratingyouth.com and at www.toniannjohnson.com. Her most recent book is *Vibrant and Clear: How to be Acne Free, Naturally.*